End-of-Life Communication in the ICU

David W. Crippen, MD

Editor

End-of-Life Communication in the ICU

A Global Perspective

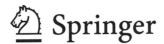 Springer

David W. Crippen, MD
University of Pittsburgh Medical Center
Pittsburgh, PA
USA

Library of Congress Control Number: 2007931623

ISBN: 978-0-387-72965-7   e-ISBN: 978-0-387-72966-4

Foreword

The specialty of intensive care was born in the polio epidemic of the 1950s. It was found that if polio patients could be ventilated by simple machines or medical students, patients could recover. The ability to maintain ventilation was important per se, but its impact was even greater in terms of the new techniques it permitted, particularly surgical. It allowed time to learn to support the circulation and, consequently, organs such as kidneys, brain, and liver, although permitting the emergence of hitherto undescribed diseases such as acute respiratory distress syndrome (ARDS).

In the early days of intensive care, charismatic enthusiasts in many countries carried the specialty forward. Although travel was long and arduous, they became personal friends and acquaintances and many of the original bright ideas were passed on in bars and offices and by mail. The rapidity of advance and discovery were limited by the ability to transmit information.

As the numbers of people who embraced the specialty grew, societies were formed and eventually specialty journals were published. Transmission of information improved in terms of dissemination but still was slow. Even the production of scientific papers was a tedious task. Younger doctors, comfortable in the PubMed or Ovid search era, often have little insight into the old process of searching the numerous copies of Index Medicus for a relevant paper and pursuing the literature through the references at the end of it. In the absence of word processing, each typographic error meant retyping the page.

Among the exciting changes in medicine over the last 10 years has been the way we communicate and manage information. The impact of the Internet on medical practice has been enormous. The latest medical research has become available immediately and the ability to communicate with colleagues, whether for fellowship or to seek real-time information on the management of patients, can now be carried out with ease, speed, and frequency.

Dr. Crippen's CCM-L (Critical Care Medicine-List) mailing list has become part of the lives of many intensivists. With respect to medical topics it has been a valuable resource for adding wisdom and experience to the literature, and a source of new friends. But perhaps its most exciting impact has been the real-time participation in major events that have medical implications. In particular, the access to information regarding the events of September 11, 2001, the severe acute respiratory syndrome (SARS) epidemic, and, more recently, Hurricane

Katrina in real time has certainly gone beyond anything that has appeared in the conventional media, and has enabled assistance and future planning.

There have been some who have expressed concerns about the role of medical discussion groups as they focus on opinion that may not be substantiated by science and consequently have the potential to be misleading. It seems to me a little unrealistic to suggest that experienced practitioners may not be able to distinguish between the two. However, Internet medical discussion groups tend more to be a place for helpful opinions often supported by science than science itself.

The ethical discussions on CCM-L are always stimulating. Certainly, they permit a range of opinions, based on the cultural, racial, and religious differences of the participants, which is in more depth than in local and national meetings. They emphasize that *different* and *correct* are not synonyms. The application to ethical issues such of diverse opinions help us all to understand the thought processes involved with these problems and to understand the way of thinking of distant colleagues.

This is the second book from Dr. Crippen in which the opinions on ethical problems are gathered largely from CCM-L members. The first was a stimulating read and an insight into the beliefs of people in other countries. Such information and kindly contemplation of the ideas of others makes us all better people.

It is interesting, however, that this information appears in a printed book. With the rapid electronic publishing rates that occur today, books, like written letters, may become a thing of the past in terms of trade and professional literature. Whether this new form of communication efficiency will replace the aesthetic value of the printed word and written letter is not known. There is surely a place for both. The written word remains for many a treasured possession to be revisited in places other than the work able. I congratulate the "lurkers" of CCM-L for their endeavors in both arenas.

Malcolm Fisher
Sydney, 2007

Preface

End-of-life issues in critical care medicine continue to confound and perplex medical consumers and physicians alike. In my first volume, I used the power of the Internet to survey the emerging global village of healthcare providers as to the contrast between their treatment preferences in end-of-life care and their capability to do so within their social and cultural structure. That discourse demonstrated a striking consensus within the international medical community, but radically different methods of accomplishing goals.

In this the second inquiry into global practices, I have again queried the global medical village on communication issues that impact the formulation of treatment care plans for patients at the end of life in intensive care units. This second volume further elucidates multinational patient and family perceptions and preferences as healthcare consumers. We then analyze how those interactions impact global healthcare delivery. This volume provides a unique insight into the mechanisms of health care in the emerging global village.

David W. Crippen, MD

Contents

Contributors

Robert M. Arnold, MD
Professor of Medicine, University of Pennsylvania, Pittsburgh, PA, USA

Richard Burrows, MB BCh (Dublin) FCA(SA)
Department of Anaesthetics, University of KwaZulu-Natal, Durban, South Africa

Donald B. Chalfin, MD, MS, FCCM
Chief Medical Officer, Analytica International & Associate Professor of Medicine, Albert Einstein College of Medicine, New York, NY, USA

David W. Crippen, MD, FCCM
Associate Professor, University of Pittsburgh Medical Center, Department of Critical Care Medicine, and Medical Director, Neurovascular Critical Care, Presbyterian University Hospital, Pittsburgh, PA, USA

Mike Darwin
Independent Critical Care Consultant, Ash Fork, Arizona, USA

Anthony L. DeWitt, RRT, CRT, JD
Attorney, Bartimus, Frickleton, Robertson & Gorny, PC, Jefferson City, MO, USA

Ilene L. Dillon, MSW
Licensed Clinical Social Worker, CEO, Emotionalpro, Kentfield, CA, USA

Justin Engleka, MSN, CRNP, MBA
Director of Professional Services, Cedars Community Hospice, Monroeville, PA, USA

Robert A. Fink, MD
Clinical Professor, Department of Neurological Surgery, University of California, San Francisco, San Francisco, CA, USA

Malcolm Fisher, AO, MBCHB, MD, FJFCM, FRCA
Professor, Intensive Care Unit, Royal North Shore Hospital, Sydney, Australia

Satoru Hashimoto, MD
Clinical Professor, Department of Anesthesiology and Intensive Care, Kyoto
Prefectural University of Medicine, Kyoto, Japan

Richard Eric Hodgson, MB, ChB(Hons)
Department of Anaesthesia, Addington Hospital and University of
KwaZulu-Natal, Durban, South Africa

Phil Hopkins, PhD, MB, BS, MRCP, FRCA
ICU Consultant, Department of Critical Care, Kings College Hospital,
London, UK

Leslie Beckhart Jenal, JD, MA
Instructor, Bioethics, Department of Religious Studies, Mount St. Mary's College,
Los Angeles, CA, USA

Farhad N. Kapadia, MD
Departments of Medicine and Critical Care, Hinduja Hospital, Mumbai,
India

Antonios Liolios, MD
Attending Physician, Intensive Care, Universite Catholique de Louvain,
Saint Lue-Hospital, Brussels, Belgium

Nicholas Macartney, MBBS, FRCA
Consultant Intensivist, Intensive Care Unit, Chase Farm Hospital, Enfield, UK

Mark A. Mazer, MD
Clinical Associate Professor and MICU Director, Department of Pulmonary
and Critical Care Medicine, East Carolina University, The Brody School of
Medicine, Greenville, NC, USA

Ted L. Rice, BS, MS, FASHP, BCPS
Associate Professor, Department of Pharmacy and Therapeutics, University
of Pittsburgh School of Pharmacy, Pittsburgh, PA, USA

Amy Roach, RN, MSN, CCRN, CNRN
Neuroscience Clinical Nurse Specialist, Department of Nursing, University
of Pittsburgh Medical Center – Presbyterian Hospital, Pittsburgh, PA, USA

Aviel Roy-Shapira, MD
Senior Staff Surgeon, Critical Care, Soroka University Medical Center,
Beer Sheva, Israel

Amy Seligman, RN, BSN, CNRN
Primary Nurse Care Coordinator, Trauma Intensive Care Unit, University of
Pittsburgh Medical Center–Presbyterian Hospital, Pittsburgh, PA,USA

Stephen Streat, BSc, MB, ChB, FRACP
Intensivist, Department of Critical Care Medicine, Auckland City Hospital,
Auckland, New Zealand

Claudia V.M. Teles, MD, TE AMIB
Intensivist and Haematologist of Lamina Laboratories in Procardiaco Hospital, Rio de Janeiro, Brazil

Dan R. Thompson, MD
Associate Professor of Surgery and Anesthesiology, Alden March Bioethics Institute, Albany Medical College, Albany, NY, USA

Errington C. Thompson, MD
Trauma/Critical Care Surgeon, Department of Trauma Services, Mission Memorial Hospital, Asheville, NC, USA

Jean-Louis Vincent, MD, PhD
Head, Department of Intensive Care, Erasme University Hospital, Brussels, Belgium

Randy S. Wax, MD, MED. FRCPC
Assistant Professor, Interdisciplinary Division of Critical Care Medicine, Department of Medicine, University of Toronto, Toronto, Ontario, Canada

Leslie M. Whetstine, PhD
Assistant Professor of Philosophy, Walsh University, North Canton, OH, USA

Brain Wowk, PhD
Senior Scientist, 21st Century Medicine, Inc., Rancho Cucamonga, CA, USA

Arino Yaguchi, MD
Department of Intensive Care Medicine, Erasme Hospital, Free University of Brussels, Brussels, Belgium

Introduction

> Words are, of course, the most powerful drug
> used by mankind.
>
> —Rudyard Kipling

The world is composed of multiple, diverse populations of different race, culture, and religion. Increasingly, these populations are mixing and intermingling, both physically with faster and cheaper air travel, and mentally via communication systems, including the Internet. Knowledge of other countries, cultures, and continents can enrich society, but can also harbor conflict and tension as different peoples struggle to understand each other without losing their own identity. In 1962, Marshall McLuhan already envisaged that new electronic interdependence would recreate the world in the image of a global village.[1] The intensive care "fraternity" is little different. Intensive care medicine has grown immensely since the early days following the polio epidemics in the 1960s, but has developed in a somewhat haphazard manner until relatively recently, when some attempt at uniformity of training has emerged at the national and international level. Intensive care doctors (*intensivists*) also come from different cultures and have different religious beliefs and backgrounds and different academic and specialty experience. Intensive care medicine is, therefore, practiced differently in different countries and even in different institutions within the same country depending on broad differences in local culture and custom, but also on the individual doctors manning the unit.

But although we may have different approaches and attitudes to the way in which we practice intensive care medicine, which can result in heated debate and disagreement, our ultimate aim is the same: to treat the critically ill patient to the best of our ability within the limitations of available equipment and facilities. Over recent years, with the development and availability of electronic mass media, intensivists are increasingly seeing themselves as part of a bigger picture, part of a global network of physicians, a global village within the wider medical world, where sharing information, data, and practices across national and international boundaries can provide benefit for us and also for our patients.

This global vision has seen fruit in several large international studies, which have been conducted by collaboration among intensivists from centers worldwide, brought together by improved international communication systems. International groups of intensivists have also been brought together to develop guidelines for various disease processes, including sepsis.[2] However, while clinical practice will vary at a national and international level due to diversity in medical training, facilities, funding, legal constraints, physician preferences, etc., the impact of diverse cultural and religious backgrounds is perhaps greatest when faced with ethical dilemmas, an all too common event in today's intensive care unit.

In an earlier book,[3] Dr. David Crippen and colleagues drew together an international group of intensivists using the Internet to discuss how the global village deals with the clinical treatment of ICU patients at the end of life. In the present volume, the focus is on communication — how doctors communicate with patients and families about end-of-life issues, and how this aspect of intensive care practice differs, or doesn't, at an international level. Several studies have addressed international differences in end-of-life care, in general, in the intensive care unit. From these studies, differences in how, how much, and with whom we communicate in the end-of-life situation can be identified. Within Europe, an ethical questionnaire answered by 504 intensive care unit physicians from 16 western European countries reported that doctors from the southern European countries of Italy, Greece, and Portugal were less likely to involve the patient and the family in decisions about end-of-life care than doctors from United Kingdom and Switzerland.[4] More recently, in the large ETHICUS study involving 4248 patients from 37 European intensive care units in 17 countries, it was noted that 95% of patients lacked decisionmaking capacity at the time of the end-of-life decision and that patient's wishes were known in only 20% of cases.[5] End-of-life decisions were discussed with the family in 68% of cases, again more commonly in the northern than central or southern European countries. Nurses were also more commonly involved in these decisions in northern European countries.[6] These results from international studies are supported by data from national studies. In France, the family was actively involved in decision making in 44% of cases and only informed in 13%.[7] In Spain, 28.3% of decisions to withdraw or withhold therapy at the end of life were made without informing the family.[8] In Portugal, Cardoso and colleagues reported that less than 11% of intensivists involve patients' relatives in end-of-life decisions, with 15% involving nurses in these decisions, although many more felt nurses and families should be involved.[9] In Italy,[10] 82% of withdrawal/withhold decisions were made by the medical team, with the involvement of nurses in just 13%; interestingly, 56% of Italian physicians said they would never involve a patient in such decisions, even if competent, and 19% of physicians said the close family were never involved in such decisions. In Sweden,[11] the general public, nurses, and physicians were asked how they would react to end-of-life decision making in different case scenarios. In the case of a conscious, competent patient, almost 50% of the general public felt that the patient should make the decision to withhold/withdraw therapy with no input from the physician, and, interestingly, 31% of the nurses and 8% of the doctors felt the same. For an unconscious patient, 73% of the general public and 70% of the nurses felt the decision should be made jointly by the physician and family; 61% of the physicians felt they should be the sole decision maker in this case.[11] Moving further afield, a recent study from Lebanon indicated that the nursing staff was not involved in 26%

of the decisions to limit care, and families were not involved in the decision in 21% of cases.[12]

In North America, patient autonomy is considered as playing a more important role in end-of-life decisions than in Europe, where medical opinion is more central.[13] In a very recent study, Yaguchi and colleagues used e-mail to survey the attitudes of intensivists to a case scenario of a patient in a vegetative state due to anoxic encephalopathy after cardiac arrest. A total of 1961 intensivists from 21 countries answered the survey. Fewer respondents in the United States and Canada replied that they would make the decision alone or just with other physicians (27% and 29%, respectively) than in other geographic regions (Europe, Australia, Turkey, Brazil, Japan). Respondents from Northern and Central Europe replied more often than other areas that they would involve nurses in such discussions, particularly in the United Kingdom, in France, and in Switzerland, where 80% of doctors involved nurses. Less than 40% of respondents from Southern Europe replied that they would involve nurses ($p > 0.0001$ vs. Northern or Central Europe), and percentages for Turkey (41%), Brazil (38%), Japan (39%), and the United States (29%) were similarly low.[13] Hence, although there seems to be universal agreement that a shared approach to end-of-life decision making, involving the caregiver team and patient/patient surrogate, is desirable,[14] and despite increased openness and discussion of these issues and the publication of guidelines and recommendations,[14-16] striking international and individual differences remain.

Multiple reasons can be proposed to explain these differences, including differences in culture and laws at a global level and differences in age, religion, sex, training, and experience at a more individual level. Interestingly, in a recent survey of physicians (not just intensivists) involved in end-of-life care in six European countries and Australia, Miccinesi and colleagues[17] reported that country was the strongest determinant of physician attitude to end-of-life decisions, although the individual physician characteristics of age, religious beliefs, sex, and previous experience with dying patients were also strong determinants.

This is an area of intensive care medicine where a global, one-size-fits-all approach is difficult to define, and, as suggested by Yaguchi and colleagues,[13] "best practice" in end-of-life care could perhaps be best defined by creating a set of basic universal ethical standards but allowing for more specific aspects, for example, the exact technique of withdrawing, etc., to be adapted to individual countries and situations. Exploring the differences among countries and individuals and the reasons behind these differences is important to enable us to determine which aspects can be considered globally definable and which must be left to individual countries, regions, or cultures.

Books such as this, and instruments such as CCM-L (Critical Care Medicine-List) mailing list, encourage physicians from all corners of the globe to discuss the important and often difficult ethical challenges that we all face on a regular basis. Effective communication between diverse populations of doctors in real time will improve understanding within the global intensivist village, which will ultimately assist in our end-of-life discussions with patients and families.

Jean-Louis Vincent and Arino Yaguchi

References

1. McLuhan HM. The Gutenberg galaxy: the making of typographic man. Toronto: University of Toronto Press; 1962.
2 Dellinger RP, Carlet JM, Masur H, et al. Surviving sepsis campaign guidelines for management of severe sepsis and septic shock. Crit Care Med 2004;32:858–873.
3. Crippen D, Kilcullen JK, Kelly DF, eds. Three patients - international perspective on intensive care at the end of life. Boston: Kluwer Academic Publishers; 2002.
4. Vincent JL. Forgoing life support in Western European intensive care units: the results of an ethical questionnaire. Crit Care Med 1999;27:1626–1633.
5. Cohen S, Sprung C, Sjokvist P, et al. Communication of end-of-life decisions in European intensive care units. Intensive Care Med 2005;31:1215–1221.
6. Benbenishty J, Ganz FD, Lippert A, et al. Nurse involvement in end-of-life decision making: the ETHICUS Study. Intensive Care Med 2006; 32(1):15–17.
7. Ferrand E, Robert R, Ingrand P, Lemaire F. Withholding and withdrawal of life support in intensive-care units in France: a prospective survey. French LATAREA Group. Lancet 2001;357:9–14.
8. Esteban A, Gordo F, Solsona JF, et al. Withdrawing and withholding life support in the intensive care unit: a Spanish prospective multi-centre observational study. Intensive Care Med 2001;27:1744–1749.
9. Cardoso T, Fonseca T, Pereira S, Lencastre L. Life-sustaining treatment decisions in Portuguese intensive care units: a national survey of intensive care physicians. Crit Care 2003;7:R167–R175.
10. Giannini A, Pessina A, Tacchi EM. End-of-life decisions in intensive care units: attitudes of physicians in an Italian urban setting. Intensive Care Med 2003;29:1902–1910.
11. Sjokvist P, Nilstun T, Svantesson M, Berggren L. Withdrawal of life support–who should decide? Differences in attitudes among the general public, nurses and physicians. Intensive Care Med 1999;25:949–954.
12. Yazigi A, Riachi M, Dabbar G. Withholding and withdrawal of life-sustaining treatment in a Lebanese intensive care unit: a prospective observational study. Intensive Care Med 2005;31:562–567.
13. Levy MM. Evaluating our end-of-life practice. Crit Care 2001;5:182–183.
14. Carlet J, Thijs LG, Antonelli M, et al. Challenges in end-of-life care in the ICU. Statement of the 5th International Consensus Conference in Critical Care: Brussels, Belgium, April 2003. Intensive Care Med 2004;30:770–784.
15. Cohen SL, Bewley JS, Ridley S, Goldhill D. Guidelines for limitation of treatment for adults requiring intensive care. Available at: http://www.ics.ac.uk/downloads/LimitTreatGuidelines2003.pdf. Accessed December 2005.
16. Truog RD, Cist AF, Brackett SE, et al. Recommendations for end-of-life care in the intensive care unit: the Ethics Committee of the Society of Critical Care Medicine. Crit Care Med 2001;29:2332–2348.
17. Miccinesi G, Fischer S, Paci E, et al. Physicians' attitudes towards end-of-life decisions: a comparison between seven countries. Soc Sci Med 2005;60:1961–1974.

1
Multinational Perspectives on End-of-Life Issues in the Intensive Care Unit

The United States

Mark A. Mazer

Communication skills are paramount to the successful and humane practice of critical care medicine. By definition, patients admitted to the critical care unit have a substantial likelihood of dying, therefore open and honest communication with the patient and significant others must begin from the earliest moments of intensive care. The Study to Understand Prognoses and Preferences for Outcomes and Risks of Treatments (SUPPORT) was conducted in five large American teaching hospitals.[1] This study demonstrated that physicians, patients, and families often do not communicate well concerning end-of-life issues. Further, the active intervention of a trained intermediary to enhance communication did little to improve the end-of-life experience, and many patients who would have otherwise wished to forgo resuscitation spent time comatose or mechanically ventilated prior to death.

Patients and their significant others must be treated in a holistic sense. It is impossible and impractical to neglect the needs of the significant others while caring for the critically ill patient. Not only the patient, but also his entire cosmos is mortally threatened by critical illness. To treat the patient while neglecting the needs of his entourage can only sow the seeds of mistrust and foster an inimical psychological and emotional climate. Thus, from the very beginning of the patient's sojourn in the intensive care unit (ICU), the clinician and the members of the multidisciplinary healthcare team must forge bonds of trust with the patient and the significant members of his personal universe.[2] Belated attempts to open a dialogue with the patient's significant others at the penultimate moments of life, when the patient is clearly dying and further treatment futile, are bound to be met with skepticism if not hostility.

Members of the multidisciplinary critical care team must strive to create an environment of open communication. The benefits of proactive communication include appropriately directed aggressive efforts towards those likely to benefit, while instituting palliative care for those who are dying and unlikely to recover.[2,3] From the outset an attempt must be made to become acquainted with the patient as a person and to understand his values. Allowing family

1

and friends to talk about their loved one helps to lessen their anxiety, and affords them the opportunity to lend assistance to the healthcare team. Often they have been aiding the patient for quite some time prior to the onset of critical illness, and to be shunned or excluded during the most uncertain and grave moments can only provoke sentiments of envy, jealousy, and hostility towards the healthcare providers. We permit select significant others to be present during bedside rounds, incorporate their opinions as we develop care plans, and otherwise update them several times per day about the condition of their loved one. Further, we are firm believers in the practice and benefits of family presence during cardiopulmonary resuscitation.[4-6]

Many critical care practitioners do not communicate well with patients and their families. During family conferences physicians tend to dominate the conversations, whereas family members are frustrated because they are not allowed enough opportunity to express themselves.[7,8] If the family is embraced from the outset, communicated with frequently and honestly, and allowed to participate in concert with the medical team, then the chances of serious conflicts at the close of life will be minimized.[1]

The stages of coping with death and dying have been well studied and described.[9] Not only the patient, but also the family and significant others must pass through the stages of denial and isolation, anger, bargaining, depression, and final acceptance. The astute critical care practitioner must treat not only the patient, but must also lend support to those suffering along with the patient. It is important to ensure that the family unit is able to carry on in a healthy and functional manner after death of the patient. The intensivist must take sufficient time to become acquainted with the various family members, and understand the particularities of the relationships they have with the patient.

Intensivists enter the life of the patient and his family in the moment of crisis and possible death. The entrance may occur at different phases of a patient's illness, and this needs to be assessed. The crisis may be unexpected and catastrophic, such as a devastating intracranial hemorrhage, or may occur at the end of a long and protracted illness, such as nosocomial pneumonia in a patient undergoing chemotherapy for cancer. Understandably, the patient and his family may be at different stages of acceptance of death and dying upon admission to the ICU. In the first instance the physician may be faced with a patient and family in denial and perhaps quite angry. For example, they may furiously blame the family practitioner for inadequate control of the patient's hypertension. On the other hand they may be quite accepting, citing the patient's determined and deliberate noncompliance with his antihypertensive medicines. In the second instance the family may be quite prepared and accepting of the possible imminent death of their long-suffering loved one. Alternatively, the family may have been inadequately apprised of the true nature of the underlying disease and prognosis by the primary care team, and may feel betrayed and be quite enraged. It is incumbent upon the critical care physician to properly assess the psychodynamic terrain in a nonjudgmental manner.

While in the ICU, the family and the patient may pass through the various stages of coping and grief at different moments in time.[9] As the stay in the

ICU prolongs, and the patient eventually becomes moribund, the family and the patient may become emotionally desynchronized. The heavily sedated, irreversibly dying patient, with vital signs supported only by a plethora of technological intervention, has probably already accepted death, is at peace, and is already quite distanced from his loved ones. Whereas the patient may have peacefully accepted the inevitable, his family members may still be wracked with sentiments of abandonment, guilt, and anger. Further, they may be suffering greatly from malaise engendered by their impotence to successfully intervene to reverse an irreversible situation.

This is the moment of greatest challenge for the critical care team, when they have given up hope, wish to discontinue life support, and allow the patient to pass on with peace, comfort, and dignity. If the family is still in a stage of denial, anger, or bargaining, then there is the potential for serious conflict. At this point the family must become the focus of attention, and be treated with the utmost kindness, compassion, and understanding. The patient will be best served if the physician gauges the family's needs and does not become an antagonist, but rather remains calm and nonjudgmental.

Often family members will express feelings of guilt concerning the imminent death of their loved one. They may feel that they have not done enough, acted quickly enough, or given enough of themselves in an effort to save their loved one. Guilt can also be due to unkind thoughts or wishes towards the loved one, and there may be a longing for exoneration. Others may feel hostility at the thought of separation and feel guilty about this anger. The physician must accept that hostility, anger, rage, and guilt-assuaging behavior may be directed toward the healthcare providers. One should allow the family to freely express these emotions and sentiments, as it is part of their healing process. It is best to allow them to grieve the anticipated loss of their loved one, and to express anger and guilt, so they may enter the final stage of peaceful acceptance.[9]

One must embrace the concept that the patient and his significant others are to be treated concomitantly from the very beginning of a critical illness.[2,3,7,8] The instances of well-intended but misguided requests to continue obviously futile medical therapy must be carefully examined to understand the genesis of the request. Failure to proactively communicate is frequently the basis of disagreement when the healthcare team comes to the unilateral decision to discontinue aggressive care. If the family and healthcare team have not been communicating openly and honestly from the start, then this wound must be acknowledged and healed. With death looming inevitably on the horizon, it is a most unpropitious moment to make amends. At this juncture it may be very difficult to commence earnest but overdue communication in an effort to elicit the family's support to curtail aggressive care. The physician must be extremely humble and forthright in accepting responsibility for this failure, and strive to gain the trust and respect of the family. Only in this manner, when the physician is eventually recognized as a trustworthy advocate rather than an antagonist, will the family accept the inevitable and let go of their loved one.

The critical care practitioner must remain calm, nonjudgmental, and maintain a sense of equanimity as the anguished family transits through the sequential stages of coping with the imminent death of their loved one. We must fulfill our fiduciary responsibility as holistic healers, and never give in to the temptation to become adversaries. Without adversaries, there can be no conflict, only peace, and this is what is best for the dying patient and his significant others.

References

1. The SUPPORT Principal Investigators. A controlled trial to improve care for seriously ill hospitalized patients: The Study to Understand Prognoses and Preferences for Outcomes and Risks of Treatments (SUPPORT). JAMA 1995;274:1591–1598.
2. Prendergast T, Puntillo K. Withdrawal of life support: intensive caring at the end of life [Perspectives on Care at the Close of Life: Clinician's Corner]. JAMA 2002;288:2732–2740.
3. Lilly C, Sonna L, Haley J, Massaro F. Intensive communication is associated with durable reductions in intensive care unit length of stay and reduced mortality in critically ill adult medical patients. Crit Care Med 2003;31:S394–S399.
4. Doyle CJ, Post H, Burney R, Maino J, Keefe M, Rhee KJ. Family participation during resuscitation: an option. Ann Emerg Med 1987;16:673–675.
5. Hanson C, Strawser D. Family presence during cardiopulmonary resuscitation: Foote Hospital emergency department's nine-year perspective. J Emerg Nurs 1992;18:104–106.
6. Mazer M. Witnessed cardiopulmonary resuscitation: the public's perception. Crit Care 2004;8(Suppl 1):P296.
7. McDonagh J, Elliott T, Engelberg R, et al. Family satisfaction with family conferences about end-of-life care in the intensive care unit: increased proportion of family speech is associated with increased satisfaction. Crit Care Med 2004;32:1484–1488.
8. Azoulay E, Chevret S, Leleu G, et al. Half the families of intensive care unit patients experience inadequate communication with physicians. Crit Care Med 2000;28:3044–3049.
9. Ross, E. On death and dying. New York: Macmillian; 1970.

Canada

Randy S. Wax

Canadian health care is dominated by overriding themes that influence most interactions between patients, family members, and healthcare teams. Many of these themes are applicable to situations related to end-of-life care for patients in the intensive care unit (ICU). Health care in Canada is a provincial responsibility. National principles must be followed by the provinces to ensure steady transfer of federal funds for health care, and are delineated in the Canada Health Act. The details and history of these principles have been reviewed and are available online for those interested.[1] The principle of public administration requires all provinces to administer public healthcare plans through a nonprofit single administrative body. The principle of comprehensiveness requires provincial health plans to insure all services that are "medically necessary," although the definition of necessity differs between provinces. The principles of universality and accessibility are meant to ensure that all members of the public within each province can access similar insured services, regardless of geographic location, and free from discrimination based on financial or health status. Private health care is limited in Canada, and would rarely be relevant to life-threatening situations such as those conditions requiring ICU care. Thus, public expectations for health care assume free and unlimited access to "necessary" care, and represent a basic right of citizenship.

Respect for religious and cultural differences in approach to end-of-life planning may also be protected by the national Charter of Rights and Freedoms.[2] However, the Charter has not been extensively used in handling individual legal cases related to end-of-life care, and therefore how it may influence decision making in futile cases is unclear.

There is strong support of the concept of autonomy in end-of-life planning for patients in a Canadian ICU. The emphasis on respecting autonomy, even at the expense of beneficence, has been described in one study comparing Canadian physician attitudes with other countries.[3] An influential recent court decision in Ontario has reinforced that autonomy may override other factors when dealing with potentially futile situations.[4] In this case, despite what were considered to be reasonable and well-meaning attempts by an intensivist to limit future life support in a patient with irreversible and progressive neurological impairment, the court found that the religious beliefs of the patient expressed by substitute decision makers took precedence.

There would be no direct financial burden on the families of patients related to the use of continued critical care in futile situations, and thus financial considerations would not typically influence preferences for choosing a more or less aggressive treatment approach to end-of-life care. Although the scarcity of critical care resources is on the mind of most Canadian intensivists, they are discouraged from allowing concern for systemwide issues influence the end-of-life care plan for individual patients. Canadian physicians are more likely to suggest withdrawal of life support in seemingly futile situations when advance directives or substitute decision makers are not available, compared with physicians in other countries.[5]

Proceeding with development of an end-of-life plan for a Canadian patient with irreversible multiorgan failure can be a complex process. Palliation in the form of relief of pain and anxiety would take place in all cases, regardless of continuation or withdrawal of life support. Discontinuation of life support would require a conversation with the patient if possible; however, most cases would only allow discussion with substitute decision makers such as family members. Patients may designate their substitute decision maker through an advance directive; however, failing this each province has a specific process for identifying a prioritized list of possible decision makers based on closeness of family relationship. In some cases, where no predesignated or related decision makers are available, a government-appointed advocate is arranged. Discussions may include only the designated substitute decision maker (e.g., spouse), but frequently also include extended family members and invited friends.

Meetings to discuss end-of-life plans for a patient with irreversible multiorgan failure would usually start with a review of the patient's condition, all of the efforts made to reverse their problems, and a discussion of the likely course with continued life support. Family members would be reassured that aggressive palliative measures would be continued to ensure that the patient did not suffer during the withdrawal of life support, and that Canadian ICU staff are very good at providing a high quality of death.[6] Many intensivists would emphasize that life support is no longer making the patient better, but in fact is prolonging their inevitable death. Although variable, many experienced intensivists would make a clear recommendation that, from the medical team's point of view, further life support measures would not meet the goals of most patients (e.g., recover to point of going home; recover enough to interact with family members). Family members would then be asked to reflect on what has been said, and then asked to speculate on what the patient might say about continued aggressive life support under the circumstances if they were able to comment.

In many cases, patients expressed clear wishes to family members that they would not want prolonged life support in the event of an irreversible situation, and the medical team reaches a consensus with the family to withdraw life support and shift to aggressive palliation, with no further plans for resuscitation. Continuous analgesic and anxiolytic infusions would be started, regardless of the extent of neurological impairment of the patient. Although approaches to details of the withdrawal of life support vary considerably between physicians and institutions, in most cases patients would be observed in the ICU for a period of hours during the process to ensure patient comfort and to allow for some continuity of care for the sake of the family. Following withdrawal of life support, should a patient appear likely to live for an extended period, transfer to a palliative care or general medical inpatient ward would be arranged. In some hospitals, where palliative care specialists are available, they would be introduced to the family prior to transfer out of the ICU and asked to be a resource to the families and to non-ICU medical services to ensure continued comfort of the dying patient. Although many families request for patients to be taken home to die prior to or following withdrawal of life support, community resources are usually inadequate to handle the complicated logistical issues of such a request.[7]

In some cases, family members do not agree with the recommendation to withdraw life support. A Canadian ICU team would almost never unilaterally withdraw life support while the family raises objections. The first step taken would be to ensure that the family truly understands what the ICU team has explained, and to explore their reasons for refusing withdrawal of life support. Family uncertainty of the irreversibility of the patient's condition can often be resolved through more detailed explanation, additional consultation by other physicians, and occasionally through review of the case by an external intensivist as a second opinion. Religious or cultural concerns with withdrawal of life support are common, particularly in large cities in Canada with extensive multicultural and immigrant populations. In such cases, involvement of clergy or social workers familiar with the patient's background is often helpful to bridge understanding and resolve issues of conflict. While further discussion takes place, ICU teams will frequently negotiate that patients should not be resuscitated in the event of a cardiac arrest, and that life support should not be escalated in the event of clinical deterioration.

Difficult cases of disagreement between the ICU team and the family of patients with irreversible organ failure do occur despite considerable effort. In such cases, Canadian hospitals usually indicate a series of steps that must take place to attempt to resolve differences. Clinical ethics teams are often brought in as consultants to identify important issues to family members and the clinical team. Physicians may appeal to government boards to override the substitute decisionmaking capability of family members when it can be demonstrated that they are acting against the best interest of the patient or against their preexpressed wishes. Extensive and prolonged court battles to decide the fate of patients with irreversible multiorgan failure are rare, and when they do occur the patient often dies prior to any final court decisions due to progression of their disease or further complications despite continued life support.

In summary, end-of-life planning for Canadian patients with irreversible organ failure in the ICU requires consensus between the medical team and the patient or substitute decision maker. When families accept that the patient cannot recover, and that the ICU team can provide appropriate palliation, life support is usually withdrawn without extensive prolongation of death. The cost of end-of-life care, including prolonged life support in challenging cases, is not borne by family members involved in end-of-life planning, and thus does not usually influence their willingness to agree to withdrawal of life support. Patient advance directives, combined with religious and cultural beliefs, are major factors influencing the end-of-life process.

References

1. Madore O. The Canada Health Act: overview and options (94-4E). Library of Parliament Parliamentary Information and Research Service. Available at: http://www.parl.gc.ca/information/library/PRBpubs/944-3.htm. Accessed October 4, 2005.
2. Jackman M. The application of the Canadian Charter in the health care context. Health Law Rev 2001;9(2):22–27. Available at: http://www.law.ualberta.ca/centres/hli/pdfs/hlr/v9_2/jackmanfrm.pdf. Accessed October 4, 2005.
3. Bruera E, Neumann CM, Mazzocato C, Stiefel F, Sala R. Attitudes and beliefs of palliative care physicians regarding communication with terminally ill cancer patients. Palliat Med 2000;14:287–298.
4. Scardoni v. Hawryluck. CanLII 34326 (ON S.C.). 2004. Available at: http://www.canlii.org/on/cas/onsc/2004/2004onsc10339.html. Accessed October 4, 2005.
5. Yaguchi A, Truog RD, Curtis JR, et al. International differences in end-of-life attitudes in the intensive care unit: results of a survey. Arch Intern Med 2005;165:1970–1975.
6. Rocker GM, Heyland DK, Cook DJ, Dodek PM, Kutsogiannis DJ, O'Callaghan CJ. Most critically ill patients are perceived to die in comfort during withdrawal of life support: a Canadian multicentre study. Can J Anaesth 2004;51:623–630.
7. Kelley ML, Habjan S, Aegard J. Building capacity to provide palliative care in rural and remote communities: does education make a difference? J Palliat Care 2004;20:308–315.

New Zealand

Stephen Streat

New Zealand[1] is a small Pacific nation (population, 4 million), first settled from Polynesia in the mid-13th century, colonized by Britain in the 19th century, and declared independent in 1907. A covenantal treaty between the indigenous (Maori) people and the British Crown was signed in 1840. New Zealand has a long egalitarian social tradition (universal suffrage, social welfare, public health care, and education) and is a free and open society[2] that is increasingly multicultural after a Māori cultural renaissance and substantial recent immigration, particularly from Polynesia and Asia. Per capita gross domestic product (GDP) at purchasing power parity (US $23,200) is only 86% of that of the European Union and 58% of that of the United States.[3] Total health expenditure (~78% of which is government funded[4]) is 8.5% of GDP.

Intensive care medicine began early in New Zealand[5-7] but resources are scarce[8] — there are only 5.4 intensive care unit (ICU) beds per 100,000 people, similar to the United Kingdom but substantially less than in the United States and much of Europe. Only 1.7% of hospital beds are critical care beds, compared to 13% in the United States,[9] 4% in Canada, and 2.6% in Australia,[8] and only 0.09% of GDP is spent on intensive care,[8] compared to 0.56% of GDP[9] in the United States.

Almost all ICUs[8] are "closed" and in public hospitals, staffed by salaried professionals.[10] A 1:1 nurse-to-patient ratio is the accepted standard for ventilated patients,[11] but there are no nurse-extenders, respiratory therapists, or physician-assistants.

Selecting patients for admission is accepted practice and ICU admission policies commonly contain similar statements to our own:

The Intensivists believe that it is incumbent upon ourselves, and upon all senior medical staff, to be aware of the resource implications of the clinical decisions we make, and to allocate healthcare resources wisely. In making patient care decisions we take fundamental ethical principles into account, including the balance between potential good and potential harm to the patient, respect for the patient's and the family's needs and values, and equity in the use of health resources.

and

Patients most likely to benefit ... are those with reversible or potentially reversible, life threatening disorders of vital systems. In deciding who is most likely to benefit the following factors are considered: - the preceding chronic health status and quality of life, physiological reserve or biological (not chronological) age, severity of acute illness, probability of reversibility and anticipated disability. Some of these factors are often unknown and it is our philosophy to give the patient "the benefit of the doubt" under conditions of uncertainty.

Withholding and withdrawing treatment is accepted practice, informed and supported by policy documents of the Joint Faculty of Intensive Care Medicine.[12,13] There is no equivalent of the (US) concept of a "legally mandated surrogate"; relevant New Zealand legislation[14] includes a Code of Health and Disability Services Consumers' Rights ("the Code") which states:

Where a consumer is not competent to make an informed choice and give informed consent, and no person entitled to consent on behalf of the consumer is available, the provider may provide services where - a) It is in the best interests of the consumer; and b) Reasonable steps have been taken to ascertain the views of the consumer; and c) Either, - i. If the consumer's views have been ascertained, and having regard to those views, the provider believes, on reasonable grounds, that the provision of the services is consistent with the informed choice the consumer would make if he or she were competent; or ii. If the consumer's views have not been ascertained, the provider takes into account the views of other suitable persons who are interested in the welfare of the consumer and available to advise the provider.

Communication with patients and families about end-of-life issues seems relatively straightforward within such a cultural framework.

When intensive care admission is judged inappropriate we may meet with patients and families and facilitate a care plan that does not include ICU admission (but may include active treatments and also ensures that the patient is free of suffering[15]). We admit some patients to the ICU but withhold or limit certain therapies[16] (e.g., when there is severe comorbidity). We make these arrangements explicit to other involved clinicians and make the implications of this "trial of intensive treatment" clear to the family (and the patient, if appropriate).

Whenever a patient with a high-mortality condition (e.g., sepsis, traumatic brain injury) is admitted to the ICU, an intensivist and the patient's nurse formally meet with the family (self-defined and often consisting of 15–30 people) within 24 hours and subsequently on a daily basis when the course is unfavorable.

These meetings occur in a large specifically designed room in the ICU. We ensure that we are not hurried or interrupted. We eschew euphemisms or "medical jargon".[17] We explain the sequence of events up to the present, the nature of the current situation, and our immediate plans. We ensure that the family understands that the patient might die during this illness. We assure them that we are providing whatever treatment is appropriate and are also making sure that the patient does not suffer either from the illness or our treatments. We listen for comments and answer all questions honestly and fully. We seek to establish mutual understanding and trust and avoid conflict with the family by maintaining open and frank dialogue. We have not yet had to take recourse to the courts to resolve disagreements, nor has an intensivist in New Zealand yet been subject to legal redress over such an issue.

We do not prognosticate hastily but do propose withdrawal of intensive treatments when it is evident that there is either very severe central nervous system (CNS) damage[18] or relentlessly deteriorating multiple organ failure; for example, treatment was withdrawn on 66/627 patients with severe traumatic brain injury, 54/141 with hypoxic–ischemic encephalopathy, 32/244 with subarachnoid hemorrhage, and 16/145 with sepsis. We make consensus decisions with other clinicians and the family, seeking "agreement" without "asking permission." We interview the next-of-kin of all patients who die[19] and find that most have understood and accepted the process of withdrawal of treatment.[18]

References

1. Te Ara – the encyclopaedia of New Zealand. Ministry for Culture and Heritage. New Zealand Government. Available at: http://www.teara.govt.nz/en.
2. Global corruption report 2005. Transparency International. Berlin, Germany. Available at: http://www.globalcorruptionreport.org/download.html.
3. The World Factbook 2005. Washington, DC: Central Intelligence Agency. Office of Public Affairs. Available at: http://www.cia.gov/cia/publications/factbook/.
4. New Zealand Health Expenditures 2002. World Health Organization. Available at: http://www.who.int/countries/nzl/en/.
5. Spence M. The emergency treatment of acute respiratory failure. Anesthesiology 1962;23:524–537.
6. Spence M. An organization for intensive care. Med J Aust 1967;1:795–801.
7. Phillips GD, Trubuhovich RV. A record of events – the first 25 years. Carlton: Australian and New Zealand Intensive Care Society; 2001. Available at: http://www.anzics.com.au/files/history_first_25.pdf.
8. Higlett T, Bishop N, Hart GK, Hicks P. Review of intensive care resources and activity 2002/2003. Melbourne: Australian and New Zealand Intensive Care Society; 2005. Available at: http://www.anzics.com.au/admc/files/arcccr_03report.pdf.
9. Halpern NA, Pastores SM, Greenstein RJ. Critical care medicine in the United States 1985-2000: an analysis of bed numbers, use, and costs. Crit Care Med 2004;32:1254–1259.
10. Cassell J, Buchman TG, Streat S, Stewart RM. Surgeons, intensivists, and the covenant of care: administrative models and values affecting care at the end of life – updated. Crit Care Med 2003;31:1551–1557; discussion, 1557–1559.
11. Minimum standards for intensive care units. Joint Faculty of Intensive Care Medicine, Australian and New Zealand College of Anaesthetists and Royal Australasian College of Physicians. 2003. Available at: http://www.jficm.anzca.edu.au/pdfdocs/icl_2003.pdf.
12. Statement on the ethical practice of intensive care medicine. Joint Faculty of Intensive Care Medicine, Australian and New Zealand College of Anesthetists and Royal Australasian College of Physicians. 2002. Available at: http://www.jficm.anzca.edu.au/pdfdocs/ic9_2002.pdf.
13. Statement on withholding and withdrawing treatment. Joint Faculty of Intensive Care Medicine, Australian and New Zealand College of Anesthetists and Royal Australasian College of Physicians. 2004. Available at: http://www.jficm.anzca.edu.au/publications/policy/ic14_2004.htm.
14. The Health and Disability Commissioner Act 1994. Available at: http://www.hdc.org.nz/index.php.
15. Streat SJ. Illness trajectories are also valuable in critical care. BMJ 2005;330:1272.
16. Streat S, Judson JA. Cost containment: the Pacific. New Zealand. New Horizons 1994;2:392–403.
17. Cassell J. Life and death in intensive care. Philadelphia: Temple University Press; 2005.
18. Streat S. When do we stop? Crit Care Resuscitation 2005;7:227–232.
19. Cuthbertson SJ, Margetts MA, Streat SJ. Bereavement follow-up after critical illness. Crit Care Med 2000;28:1196–1201.

United Kingdom

Nicholas Macartney

The position in the United Kingdom with respect to end-of -life issues is mainly driven by the General decision of the court, not distant Medical Council (GMC) guidance, "Good Medical Practice."[1] This has been subject to recent review by the Appeal Court, following the case of Oliver Leslie Burke vs. General Medical Council.[2] Because of the GMC document, there has been little research in this area in the United Kingdom.

While this document covers many areas, one section deals with withholding and withdrawing care. Several parts of it can be seen as determining the actions of medical staff in the United Kingdom, and show the legal differences in the United Kingdom from other parts of the world. The essence of this document is that adult competent patients have the right to refuse treatment, even where this may result in their own death. Where patients are unable to decide for themselves, it is the doctor's responsibility to decide what is in the patient's best interests, taking into account as much information as can be gleaned about the patient and the benefits and burdens of treatment. However, it is also stated that, "if a patient wishes to have a treatment that in the doctor's considered view is not clinically indicated, there is no ethical or legal obligation on the doctor to provide it."

In the judgement of the court of appeal, this was confirmed that "if a doctor concludes a treatment is not clinically indicated, he is not required to provide it to the patient, although he should offer to arrange a second opinion."

This means that when dealing with end-of-life issues in the United Kingdom, the ultimate decision lies with the medical staff, or with the patient in the event that the patient wishes treatment to be withdrawn. Family have no rights, except to express the patient's views if the patient is unable to do so, with the result that when one enters into a meeting with the family, the family do not have the right to overrule the doctors.

Although the culture is changing, there still remains an element, particularly among the elderly, that "doctor knows best," and because of the UK system with family doctors building up long-term relationships with families, family members often have experienced past episodes of care within the same hospital, so are more likely to have some trust for the medical staff, as demonstrated by opinion poll evidence of trust in doctors. This helps to bring an element of trust and mutual respect into the meeting.

With this background, all intensive care units (ICUs) try to establish close relationships with relatives as soon as possible. Within the limits of confidentiality, families are kept informed of the patient's progress. In my unit, and in many others, the consultant (specialist) meets with relatives to tell them in person what has happened, what might happen, and to give an assessment of likely outcome. In my practice I will tell the family that the ICU mortality in the United Kingdom is about 25%, and if asked will attempt to estimate the patient's risk of death, based on our audit results. This early, frank discussion establishes the relationship, makes the family aware of how sick the patient is, and helps with future meetings.

Having had these discussions in the earlier part of the stay, in the event of end-of-life discussions, the family is often well aware of the situation. Frequently they have come to accept that their relative is not improving, and the family may, in fact, raise the subject of withdrawal themselves. In these discussions, the most important requirements are openness, honesty, and answering as fully as possible any questions the family may have. From a practical point of view, one should allow sufficient time, which may easily exceed an hour. In the United Kingdom, the defense organizations always advocate openness, and make the point that sympathy and an apology are not an admission of liability, but are a demonstration of humanity. Explaining to the family what has happened in the ICU, explaining as best one can why a patient has not responded to treatment, and why further treatment is not going to be helpful, in a calm environment, will help the family to accept the situation. Sometimes in this situation families think that they are being asked to make decisions, but in fact they are typically being asked to recognize the inevitable. At the same time, it is important to explain that while the *treatment* part may end, the *care* part will continue unchanged. In the United Kingdom, withdrawal of artificial nutrition and hydration from a patient would only be done after a court hearing. Making an explicit statement to the family that the patient will be kept comfortable at all times, with fluids, analgesia, and other medications as required, ensuring pastoral or religious care for family and patient, and ensuring that the staff will continue to care for the patient, while attempting to allow family as much quality time as possible with their relative assists them in this time.

The other issue that has to be addressed is duration of the dying process. Families often ask how long this will take, and prediction can be very difficult. Experience assists in this area, but it is impossible to be accurate in all cases. Withdrawal of inotropes might result in death in a very short time, while a terminal wean of a patient with a hypoxic brain injury who is otherwise stable may result in death over some days. In the United Kingdom, there are very open visiting hours in the ICU, often in excess of 6 hours per day, and these are usually relaxed entirely in these circumstances so that the family is allowed to stay continuously, including during the ward rounds. If bed pressure allows, it is better to allow patients and family to remain in the ICU, rather than undergo the unedifying process of discharge to die elsewhere in a ward, in an environment that is unfamiliar to the family, with nurses who have not met the patient before.

In summary, in the United Kingdom the legal position is that the doctors are able to make the final decision, subject to review by the courts, which usually are in agreement with the medical staff. As a result of this, one is able to have a detailed discussion with family, secure in the knowledge that the best interests of the patient will be paramount, and decisions are subject to decision of the court, not distant relatives.

References

1. http://www.gmc-uk.org/guidance/good_medical_practice/index.asp.
2. http://www.lawreports.co.uk/WLRD/2005/CACIV/julf1.5.htm.

Communicating to Family: The Israeli Perspective

Aviel Roy-Shapira

Israel is largely an immigrant state. As a result, we have to deal with a large cultural diversity. The predominant Jewish population is divided into several very distinct segments: Ultraorthodox are a small but vocal minority. The moderate orthodox outnumber the former group, but tend to follow their teachings on end-of-life issues. The majority of the Jewish population is nonreligious, but many of these consider themselves traditional. They observe some rules and disregard others. The latter group also tends to follow the ultraorthodox on end-of-life decisions. About 40% of the population is truly secular. The latter group, which by and large is also the best educated and has the highest income, tend to follow general humanistic principles about end-of-life decisions.

The Israeli legislature has traditionally avoided addressing end-of-life issues. Law does not define death. There is only a passing remark in the vital statistics law that states that a doctor who determines the death of a person must report it.

Determining death by neurological criteria is permitted, based on a Ministry of Health directive, which specifies the requirements. The legal basis for the directive is flimsy, but it has never been challenged. Jewish Law[a] requires cessation of breathing to determine death. Several rabbinical authorities have therefore accepted a positive apnea test as a sign of death. But it is not simple, as we shall see.

Israeli patients' bill of rights allows patients to refuse treatment. There is however an ongoing legal debate about withdrawal of treatment once started. There, district courts have ruled several times on specific cases, mostly amyotropic lateral sclerosis (ALS) patients, that withdrawal is permissible. However, the attorney general never appealed to the Supreme Court, so there is no binding precedence, and each case is judged separately. A recent case of a patient in a persistent vegetative state (PVS) is now before the Supreme Court, and many of us eagerly await the outcome.

The withdrawal of ventilation is considered by the media and the public to be euthanasia, a dirty word in Israel. Most Israelis, including most doctors, do not see the difference between withdrawing life support at the request of the patient (or surrogate) and withdrawing it because someone else considers the patient's life not worth living. Consequently all withdrawals are immediately compared with the Nazi euthanasia program.

---

[a] Jewish Law (with a capital L) or Halacha in Hebrew is a loosely defined code of laws and rules of conduct which is interpreted by rabbis, and is derived from Talmudic teaching. The interpretation always relies on precedence, and there are codified methods of drawing analogies, if there is no precedence to rely on. It has no legal standing in Israel (except on marital issues) but is all important for the orthodox.

Although in Jewish Law the sanctity of life has overwhelming importance — it allows you to break any rule in order to preserve life — it has several ways of going around it. For example, the Talmud says that if someone in the yard is hacking wood, and the noise impedes the soul of dying person to depart, one must go out and ask the wood hacker to stop, so that the soul can depart in peace.

One might extend this to a ventilator, but rabbinical authorities have refused to do so. However, the rabbinical authorities were under great pressure to provide a means of withdrawing treatment for obviously hopeless cases. The solution they found was while stopping treatment is forbidden, modifying it or renewing it if stopped for a different reason is not required.

Consequently, an acceptable method of withdrawing life support is to stop making any treatment adjustments. In a study of this method, all ventilated patients where treatment adjustments were stopped died within 48 hours.[1]

Another proposed alternative is to convert continuous treatment into discrete by placing timers on ventilators. This is religiously acceptable, but the technology is still under development. The timers would be set to turn the ventilator off after a preset number of days. Both of these alternatives are endorsed by the most prominent Halachic rule makers in the ultraorthodox communities, and are therefore also accepted by the more moderate orthodox and the traditional.

By law, the wishes of family members regarding medical care decisions have no impact. The next of kin cannot consent or refuse medical care for their relatives. They may do so only if a court granted them a legal guardian status. Moreover, a living will or durable power of attorney is not a binding legal instrument. There is a legislative initiative to change this, but the religious parties oppose it, and the measure has not been passed by parliament.

As a consequence of this situation, the physicians make the decision to terminate care, always based on futility, and we merely notify the family members. Only when the relatives come forward with evidence that the patient did not want treatment in this situation, care may be terminated at the initiative of the patient, at the discretion of the attending physician or ICU director.

We need a court order to stop the ventilator, except when death by neurological criteria has been pronounced. Termination really means that we stop making adjustments, and do not renew vasopressors.

The most common problem is that adult children request aggressive measures for their elderly terminally ill parents, even when they know the patients themselves would not have wished it. One Israeli study[2] found that 50% of adult children of terminally ill geriatric patients claimed to know what their parent wanted, but requested that aggressive care continue nevertheless.

An illustrative case occurred recently when shrapnel to the head wounded a girl during a terrorist attack. Death by neurological criteria was established, and the ICU attending physician proposed organ donation. The family, who were orthodox, refused. They also refused to allow a shut down. They involved several prominent rabbis and the press. Hospital administration ordered that the body should be kept on life support. The whole ordeal lasted several days, with very bad publicity.

The main problem was that the attending physician, who was worried about the reaction from the family, elected to stop the vasopressors but keep the ventilator going. This was a double message, which contributed to the turmoil. Unfortunately, this is a common attitude among Israeli critical care specialists, many of whom are reluctant to shut down.

To conclude, end-of-life decisions in Israel are complex due to the diversity of religious beliefs, and a traditional paternalistic philosophy among many physicians and critical care specialists. The orthodox community expects a paternalistic attitude, and a secular humanist physician must often do a fine balancing act.

References

1. Steinberg A. The terminally ill – ethical and Jewish perspectives. Isr J Med Sci 1996;32:601–602.
2. Sonnenblick M, Friedlander Y, Steinberg A. Dissociation between the wishes of terminally ill parents and decisions by their offspring. J Am Geriatr Soc 1993;41:599–604.

Maria and the Good Death: The Latin American View

Claudia V.M. Teles

Maria had been in our intensive care unit (ICU) for 30 days now. She was clearly dying. A uterine cervical cancer victimized her, and as she underwent chemotherapy, hemorrhagic cystitis and perforation of an intestinal wall invaded by the neoplastic cells caught her right in the nadir of chemoinduced neutropenia. She already had bone and liver metastatic disease, and probably lung infection (that was not responding to antibiotics), repeated transfusions, procoagulants, and other support measures. Despite our attempts to make the family aware of her impending death and the futility of further treatment attempts, they refused to accept it. They were extremely religious people and kept on expecting a miracle. The patient was young, 34 years old, and she was leaving a desperate husband with two small children. As bilateral ureteral obstruction and massive hemorrhage supervened, her blood urea started to rise, and we decided not to submit the patient to hemodialysis. The family questioned the decision because they wanted everything to be done, for they were still expecting a miraculous turn of events. They believed that "denying care for a human being is against Christian principles." It required a team approach to the problem and a series of discussions with several different members of the ICU team — doctors, nurses, social assistants — repeating the same words and ideas:

If we go further in the aggressive therapeutic measures, all we will do is worsen her pain and suffering. She needs rest and peace as there is nothing we can do to her but bring her more pain if we continue treatment. You must accept this and be prepared. We are doing our best to alleviate pain, and make her comfortable, so she will not be aware of what is happening. God wants no one to suffer on earth ... Suffering is part of life, however, and we are doing all we can to prevent her suffering.

When death came, her husband and parents were able to accept the fact in peace, as we managed to make them understand the concept of the "good death," through persistence and patience, with a team approach, hearing them and using their own arguments to guarantee the patient a more humane way to end her days. Understanding the religious background of the family is important in Latin America, even if the intensivist himself does not profess any religion. A wise strategy would be to be acquainted with the proper Christian logic to make people accept what cannot be changed regarding terminality.

As palliative care is only now emerging as a new specialty in Latin America, intensivists hold the burden of the terminal patients' care. Many times, a terminal patient is admitted only because the family is not used to watching someone during the passing. Very often, these patients still undergo resuscitative measures, at family request, and stay a long time in our acute care beds. The challenge in Latin America is to make lay society comprehend the concept of the Good Death, and reinforce the notion that dying without pointless painful attempts to maintain life artificially is not against Christian principles.

Implementing end-of-life care discussions among the members of the ICU team — including psychologists, social assistants, and even religious representatives in the discussions with the families — and allowing families to spend more time inside the ICU whenever it does not disturb unit routines, are the most common means found by many ICUs in Brazil, Argentina, and other Latin American countries to address communications with families on end-of-life decisions and the application of do-not-resuscitate orders, and in this regard, we do not differ from the rest of the world.[1]

New legislation is coming regarding the extent of supportive measures to be carried out in patients with doubtful prognoses. There is already a clear position of medical councils, like the São Paulo Regional Medical Council,[2,3] defending the patient's right to refuse extraordinary or painful treatments with the aim to artificially prolong life, defending patients' autonomy. These activities are creating a noticeable need to improve dialogue between the healthcare team and patients' families, in order to ensure that all the circumstances of the patient's followed, regarded that the justice principle is also preserved in the process. In Third World countries, lack of beds and resources are utmost factors when making end-of-life decisions. There is no point in prescribing extraordinary therapeutic measures for a terminal patient when there are many others with a clearly better prognosis that will be deprived of these same resources because of wrong qualitative and quantitative decisions. In a daily basis, we have to make families understand this, and find alternatives to care for terminal patients without placing them far from their beloved ones, inside an ICU, where traditionally small psychological and philosophical care is given to the anxieties of a passing human being with reserved prognosis among several other patients who still remain viable and receive most of the team's attention.

Some innovative measures in course are[4]:

- The creation of end-of-life care committees including several members of the ICU team, like physicians, nurses, social assistants, and psychologists, responsible for medical decisions and family contact.
- Implementation of end-of-life case discussions where the relatives' reactions to medical decisions are analyzed and discussed broadly, and new strategies to solve critical differences are pointed out by the ICU team members.
- Collective meetings among patient's relatives and several members of the ICU team, with the moderation of a psychologist working as a group therapy to address anxieties and frustrations from each involved part.
- Divulgation of end-of-life care brochures as part of educational programs to doctors and to the lay public.[5]

References

1. Yaguchi A, Truog RD, Randall Curtis J, et al. International differences in end-of-life attitudes in the intensive care unit: results of a survey. Arch Intern Med 2005;165:1970–1975.

2. Paulo Medical Council. Public consultation on the patient's will to refuse extraordinary support measures to prolong life. Available at: http://www.bioetica.org.br/legislacao/res_par/integra/29535_03.php.
3. Paulo Medical Council. Public consultation on cases when the physician can refuse invasive support measures and ICU admission for elderly patients. Available at: http://www.bioetica.org.br/legislacao/res_par/integra/15744_01.php.
4. Palliative care and end of life policies in Colombia. Available at: http://www.eolc-observatory.net/global_analysis/colombia_reading.htm
5. ACP-ASIM End-of-Life Care Patient Education Project. Available at: http://www.acponline.org/ethics/patient_education.htm and http://www.acponline.org/chapters/latin/br/nov2001.htm

The Greek Perspective

Antonios Liolios

> This is the Balkans — no walk in the park!
>
> —Nikos Engonopoulos, Greek poet (1907–1985)

Born and raised in Greece, I decided to do my medical residency in internal medicine in the United States and I was eventually accepted at a teaching hospital in New York City. One day during my internship, an elderly Greek man from the island of Crete was brought in by his daughter because of abdominal pain and steatorrhea. He was found to have pancreatic cancer. The daughter asked me not to disclose the diagnosis to her father to protect him from "getting upset and depressed." This was a common attitude in Greece where relatives were concerned that the cancer patient will become depressed and even commit suicide if he or she finds out the diagnosis. But what was the right thing to do in the United States? And this patient seemed depressed to begin with. The attending physician, a native of the United States, had no doubts. He ignored the daughter's pleas and eventual threats and informed the patient about the diagnosis. Later that night I visited the patient in his room. He was calm and sad. I asked him how he felt. He told me, "Son, I knew I had something bad, don't worry. I am not concerned about myself. I am concerned about my wife who will soon become a widow."

There are two major factors influencing life and death in Greece: religion and family. More than 95% of Greeks are Christian Orthodox. And while divorce rates have been increasing, family ties are very strong, and Greeks spend most of their adult lives near their parents and amongst relatives.

Orthodox Christianity encourages palliation and pain relief. The final moments of a person's life are considered very important as during these moments humans will encounter God, account for their lives, and move into eternity. Last-minute repentance and Holy Communion are considered soul saving and are offered in many Greek hospitals. Priests are often seen walking around offering Holy Communion to the gravely ill. As the primary importance of existence is the salvation of the immortal soul and its placement near Christ in heaven, aggressive life-sustaining procedures and therapeutics are not encouraged.

On the other hand, euthanasia is discouraged by the Church and is illegal in Greece. Occasionally stories of patients requesting euthanasia appear in the media, but overall such requests have not been granted.

In a large study of the views of the public and professionals in Greece, 44.3% of the 417 responders were against prolonging life with artificial means.[1] This is in accordance with the Mediterranean culture, where life is weighted primarily qualitatively and not quantitatively and remains desirable when it can be experienced with passion and dignity and not as a part of a life-sustaining machine.

Although individuality is highly praised in the Greek society, confidentiality and privacy are not the major concerns. Greeks find relief in sharing their health problems and worries and expect that others feel the same way. If you are admitted to a hospital, you may be asked questions like "What's wrong with your health?" "You look sick and pale, is your liver OK?" by your or others patients' visitors and you would be expected to answer. The Health Insurance Portability and Accountability Act (HIPAA)[2] will never flourish in Greece.

The family is usually around the terminally ill. Treating a critically ill patient often translates into treating a group of people, especially when the patient is young. Several different relatives and close friends will appear, even after years of absence, constantly requesting information and comfort.

The Church encourages organ donation and it is regarded as an act of love. In spite of that, Greeks may be very sensitive on the issue, especially when younger patients are involved. When the issue of organ donation arises, extra caution and care should be exercised. One of the fears tormenting the Greek family could be that the care of their loved one may be compromised in order to facilitate organ harvesting. The family should be made fully aware of the prognosis and options and carefully introduced to the decision for organ donation. Although there is a legal next of kin, decisions are usually made by the family as a whole. If even one family member objects this may lead to organ refusal. This should be respected and the transplant team should not persist. A disappointing fact in Greece is that although Greece holds a high rank in motor vehicle accidents in the European Union, the number of transplants is disappointing low.[3]

Withdrawing life support is not an easy task in a Greek intensive care unit (ICU). Laws surrounding the withdrawal of life support can be vague and ambiguous, allowing equivocal interpretation. The media often feature stories of physicians being sued when they withdrew or did not provide life support to a terminally ill patient. Consequently, the aim of many therapeutic interventions may be unclear, as shown in the ETHICUS study.[4]

Revealing a grave diagnosis can be a challenge, as outlined in the story at the beginning of this chapter. Cancer is a particularly scary diagnosis and many Greeks elect to hide it from their loved ones. It is not uncommon for a patient to clearly suspect his disease and the family around him or her adamantly refusing it. Often a physician will be asked to assist in this saga by calling chemotherapy "antibiotics," for example, or by even plainly denying the existence of cancer to the patient. Rarely a physician would cross the line and inform the patient about the truth, as this would cause considerable turmoil and even hostility towards him. But most importantly, most Greek physicians believe that it is often better for the patient "not to know," especially when the patient is elderly, fragile, or incapacitated.

When abroad, Greeks respect the local culture and habits and deeply appreciate the respect of their national distinctiveness. Finding a competent interpreter and a priest, if possible, will soothe the pain and relax the anxiety.

In conclusion, it appears that there are still many steps ahead that have to be taken in Greece regarding the care of the terminally ill patient. But one should not forget that individual and ethnic differences vary immensely among people and nations and they should always be carefully considered and taken into account. Universal, rigidly accepted and applied ethic rules and practices refer more to a concept of an "ethics police" where end-of-life guidelines and algorithms are followed in the same manner and with the same legal consequences as the guidelines for treating severe sepsis.[5] Admittedly, it is easier to make an ethical decision in a very homogeneous society like Greece, but with the constantly increasing immigration influx and the changing financial and political face of the Balkans, problems similar to those encountered in US ICUs are expected to arise.

Epilogue

Charalambos is a 28-year-old computer PhD student sitting next to me at the airport as I am finishing typing this article. He will soon get married and for now he is living with his parents and grandparents. We start talking about the issue of disclosing the diagnosis to cancer patients. "I would personally like to know if it happened to me," he says, "but my grandpa was diagnosed with localized prostate cancer two years ago. A big-shot doctor rushed to reveal the diagnosis to him and since then he wants to stay in bed, does not want to leave the house, and had to be admitted twice to the hospital because he wouldn't eat. Drugs and psychiatrists don't help. Telling him that he had cancer was a big mistake. That doctor was really selfish."

One has to be very careful when practicing medicine in the Balkans!

References

1. Vidalis A, Dardavessis T, Kaprinis G. Euthanasia in Greece: moral and ethical dilemmas. Aging (Milano) 1998;10:93–101.
2. Angelos P. Compliance with HIPAA regulations: ethics and excesses. Thorac Surg Clin 2005;15:513–518.
3. Mavroforou A, Giannoukas A, Michalodimitrakis E. Organ and tissue transplantation in Greece: the law and an insight into the social context. Med Law 2004;23:111–125.
4. Sprung CL, Cohen SL, Sjokvist P, et al. End-of-life practices in European intensive care units: the Ethicus Study. JAMA 2003;290:790–797.
5. Dellinger RP, Carlet JM, Masur H, et al. Surviving Sepsis campaign guidelines for management of severe sepsis and septic shock. Crit Care Med 2004;32:858–873.

The South African Perspective

Richard Eric Hodgson

South Africa is a culturally and economically diverse country that is in the process of reversing the 30-year legacy of Apartheid on the background of 300 years of European colonization and destruction of indigenous African culture. This process is being significantly hampered by two epidemics that have a profound impact on intensive care unit (ICU) service provision: human immunodeficiency virus/acquired immunodeficiency syndrome (HIV/AIDS) and trauma due to motor vehicle accidents and interpersonal violence.

The population of South Africa currently stands at 45 million people, made up of 85% black, 10% white, and 5% Indian and colored South Africans. Twenty percent of the population is covered by medical insurance and is cared for in private hospitals that consume 60% of the healthcare expenditure and employ 70% of medical specialists in South Africa. The state healthcare system consumes 40% of South Africa's healthcare expenditure and employs 30% of the medical specialists to care for 80% of the population, half of whom are not formally employed. The state healthcare system also provides the majority of training for healthcare professionals in South Africa.[1]

Critical care has been recognized as a medical subspecialty in South Africa for more than 10 years. Subspecialists from primary specialties, including medicine, surgery, pediatrics, and anesthesia were registered with the Health Professionals Council of South Africa after 2 years of training in a unit accredited by the council. For the last 3 years, a Fellowship in Critical Care has been recognized by the College of Medicine of South Africa, requiring not only 2 years of training but also the completion of a written and oral examination.

In the state sector, the majority of units are closed and led by an intensivist, as opposed to the private hospitals, where the majority of units are open with very limited intensivist input.

End-of-Life Decisions in State Intensive Care Units

The state hospital ICUs have systems in place but are limited in their effectiveness by a number of factors that include (1) staff shortages due to losses to the private hospitals and overseas; (2) resource shortages due to limited budgets for health care resulting in a decline in ICU beds to less than 1:100,000 population[2] compared with the recommendation of 5 per 100,000[3] and high demand due to the HIV/AIDS and trauma epidemics; (3) increased severity of illness due to delays in treatment at many levels, including prehospital rescue and resuscitation, emergency room management, and operative management.

State hospital ICUs typically have occupancy close to 100%, resulting in up to half of all requests for admission being turned down on the basis of no beds.[4] In South Africa, continued intensive therapy for a dying patient will prevent the resource being utilized by that patient from being used by another critically ill patient who will die without it.[5]

State hospital intensivists must make decisions to maximize the utility of the resource on the basis of triage — refusal of patients with a low likelihood of survival with or without intensive therapy — and futility — withdrawal of therapy in patients who are failing to respond to intensive interventions.

Triage decisions are typically made during a consultation between a referring clinician and the ICU physician. Triage decisions are based on criteria that are understood within the hospital and/or center but are seldom described in a written guideline. Should ICU admission be considered inappropriate by the clinicians involved, this option may or may not be raised with the family depending on the circumstances of the case.

In Durban, the ICU team makes decisions about futility with the patient's nurse as a central participant. The critical decision required of every intensivist every day on every patient treated in their ICU is whether the efforts and resources being expended on each patient are saving the patient's life or prolonging his or her death. This is not a simple or easy decision and generally requires wide consensus, not only between the treating clinicians, as demonstrated by a joint study from Cape Town and London,[6] but also between the treating clinicians, the patient, and their family.

Discussions with families in South African state ICUs may be hampered by a number of factors:

1. **Language barriers**. Interpreters are often needed and thus misinterpretation is common. This may be particularly relevant if family members have to act as interpreters.
2. **Cultural barriers**. South African society is still largely based on a paternalistic system where decisions are devolved to a senior (usually male) family member. A study from France has suggested that many family members do not want to be involved in decision making in the ICU setting.[7] There is no similar study in South Africa but the impression of state intensivists is that the results would not differ substantially.

Despite these barriers, it is still possible for families to be involved in the decisionmaking process. Every attempt is made to speak with the family as early as possible in the patient's admission, especially where death is deemed a possible, or likely, outcome. The first thing the ICU clinician does is attempt to determine what role families want to play in medical decision making. Members of the care team from a similar cultural background to the patient are invaluable in assisting in this decision, but at the same time every attempt is made to avoid placing the family in a position where they feel they are being called upon to make a decision, so that they are not left with a burden of guilt that will aggravate the trauma of their loss.

The legal validity of a medical decision to limit therapy in the face of family demands for continued treatment has not been tested in the South African ICU context. The attitude of the South African legal system may be inferred from a case in which renal dialysis was denied by a state hospital to a patient with chronic renal failure. The hospital argued that the patient did not meet the criteria for transplantation and thus had an incurable disease that should not be treated further as this would deny treatment to patients in whom cure was possible. The patient argued that his right to life guaranteed by the constitution was being infringed. The Constitutional Court found in favor of the hospital and the patient subsequently died.[8]

Cases involving medical decisions in South Africa are heard by a judge with two appropriately qualified medical practitioners acting as assessors, making an adverse finding in the face of a reasonable decision made by consensus of a number of experienced clinicians extremely unlikely.

End-of-Life Decisions in Private Intensive Care Units

Private ICUs in South Africa have facilities very similar to those in nonteaching ICUs in the United States. In terms of staffing, there are a very limited number of closed, intensivist-led ICUs in South African private hospitals. The majority of units are open and do not have an intensivist director or appropriate junior medical staffing.

The interventions applied in these ICUs, often by specialists such as cardiologists, pulmonologists, nephrologists, neurologists, etc., result in improvement in surrogate endpoints while likelihood of survival often does not improve. Efficient preservation of vital organ function over prolonged periods means that death in ICU in the United States, Europe, and Australasia is increasingly becoming a process initiated by withholding or withdrawal of organ support.[9] Clinicians in South African private ICUs are generally not specialist intensivists and thus have limited experience in initiating appropriate end-of-life discussions regarding withholding or withdrawing therapy in the ICU. Conversely, an overly optimistic attitude to outcome is very prevalent in private ICUs.

Initiation of end-of-life discussions is extremely stressful, causing continued therapy to be generally well accepted, both by hospital administrators and families. This acceptance may be reversed at the point where therapy is no longer funded. At this point hospital administrators are concerned by ongoing potential financial losses and families are concerned by generation of potentially crippling debt. This may result in requests for transfer to a state institution for continued therapy or limitation of therapy followed by transfer out of ICU or death. Transfer to a state ICU is very unlikely given the fact that the patient is already in an appropriate institution and state facilities are severely constrained.

Limitation of therapy may be appropriate but families should not be left with a burden of guilt that therapy was withheld due to their inability to pay.

Intensivists working in State institutions may have roles to play in private ICUs, including:

1. **Regular rounds**. The aim would be primarily to improve outcome for patients surviving their ICU admission, but patients in whom withdrawal may be appropriate could be identified and the necessary discussions between the care team and family initiated.
2. **Specific end-of-life consultations**. Private clinicians who identify patients in whom withdrawal may be appropriate could discuss such cases with state intensivists. The intensivist could then assist in facilitating the process of withdrawal by achieving consensus within the care team and initiating appropriate communication with the family.

Conclusion

At present, South African intensive care faces a dichotomy of a state ICU service with reasonable systems in place but severe resource constraints and a private service with adequate resources but largely deficient systems. With better communication between the services, the needs of dying patients may be more appropriately met.

References

1. http://www.southafrica.info/ess_info/sa_glance/health/health.htm.
2. Bhagwanjee S. Audit of intensive care utilisation in KwaZulu Natal: focus on King Edward VIII and Addington Hospitals. Paper presented to KZN Healthcare Task Team. 1998.
3. Lyons RA, Wareham K, Hutchings HA, Major E, Ferguson B. Population requirement for adult critical care beds: a prospective quantitative and qualitative study. Lancet 2000;355.
4. Burrows RC, Gopalan PD, Hodgson RE. DNR – The importance of the medical decision. World Congress of Intensive Care. Sydney, Australia. 2001. Free Paper 31.
5. Burrows RC, Hodgson RE. De facto gatekeeping and informed consent in intensive care. Med Law 1997;16:17–27.
6. Turner JS, Michell WL, Morgan CJ, Benatar SR. Limitation of life support: frequency and practice in a London and a Cape Town intensive care unit. Intensive Care Med 1996;22:1020–1025.
7. Azoulay E, Pochard F, Chevret S, et al., and the FAMIREA Study Group. Half the family members of intensive care unit patients do not want to share in the decision-making process: a study in 78 French intensive care units. Crit Care Med 2004;32:1832–1838.
8. Thiagraj Soobramoney vs. Minister of Health, Province of Kwazulu-Natal, South Africa. Durban Supreme Court Case Number 5846197, August 1997.
9. Manara AR, Pittman JA, Braddon FE. Reasons for withdrawing treatment in patients receiving intensive care. Anaesthesiology 1998;53:523–528.

A Perspective from India

Farhad N. Kapadia

Communication with relatives of critically ill intensive care unit (ICU) patients in India is a relatively neglected area. It poses many complexities related to the vastly heterogeneous nature of the Indian population. This heterogeneity is not only due to cultural, lingual, and religious backgrounds, but also due to difference in education and socioeconomic levels.

Unfortunately, most intensive care in India is delivered in the absence of consultant intensivists. This frequently results in multiple specialists speaking to family, often giving conflicting information and contradictory prognoses. Over the last decade, an increasing number of hospitals and ICUs are appointing consultant intensivists to manage ICU patients. It then falls upon the intensivist to ensure that some uniformity of communication is maintained and that the information given is accurate. Often the consultant intensivist is not an autonomous consultant and needs clearance from the primary consultant on what he or she discusses with the family. In other institutions, a consultant intensivist does not necessarily see all ICU patients, only those referred to him or her. In both these situations, discussions between the consultant intensivist and the relatives is colored by this unequal partnership. In institutions like the one in which I work, a consultant intensivist automatically sees all ICU admissions and speaks autonomously to relatives. As the understanding and cooperation between the intensivists and other specialists increase, the primary consultant frequently requests that the intensivist does the bulk of the communication with the family. In fact, most end-of-life discussions are done almost entirely by the consultant intensivist. Encouragingly, an increasing number of non-intensivist specialists are beginning end-of-life discussions and do not intubate (DNI) or do not resuscitate (DNR) status early in the course of hospital or ICU admission.

A typical scene in my ICU would involve a patient with a relatively straightforward medical problem requiring ICU, for example, following an acute myocardial infarction, stroke, or major surgery. Here, the primary consultant would do most or all the communication with the patient and relatives. The intensivist would further communicate with the relatives or patient if specifically requested to do so by the primary consultant or the family. In the event that the intensivist is also the primary consultant, he or she would speak to the family on a daily basis with an update of the medical situation. Quite often I choose to do this at the bedside of the patient, with the relatives present, so that the patient and the family can simultaneously grasp the situation and ask any questions.

As the patient becomes more critical, the intensivist often becomes the main consultant communicating with the family. In my first communication with family, I clarify which language we should communicate in and I ask them to identify a principle relative who should be present for daily discussions. This relative can then further explain the situation to family members not present during our discussions. I usually explain the situation as best as I can, explain what kind of life support we are using, and what we can expect over what period of time. I emphasize the serious nature of the illness and the distinct possibility of death or some other unfavorable outcome. I then encourage all present to ask me any questions they may have. I subsequently have at least one communication with the appropriate family members on a daily basis.

There are many barriers that prevent adequate communication when using this approach. Some of these are cultural while others reflect the relatively low priority given to communication with relatives. Due to space constraints, most ICUs, including mine, have no designated area for family consultation or conferences. Instead, a doctor's or nurses' office or workspace is temporarily used for this purpose. Even more unsatisfactorily, many doctor–relative communications occur in the passages or waiting areas outside the ICU, often with the doctor masking his or her impatience to hurry up with the communication so that one can get on with a busy schedule. Relatives often accept this as a fact of medical life and rarely if ever demand adequate time for communication. The next problem is of language, education, and sociocultural differences. Despite detailed and prolonged explanation from the doctor, it is not unusual to get only a limited understanding of the situation from the relatives. One needs to explain to other relatives or repeat the same facts on different occasions, until the reality of the situation is actually appreciated and understood by all. Although times are changing, it is usually expected that the main discussion be done in the presence of some male members of the family. Many doctors are reluctant to give a very bad prognosis or break bad news if only female relatives are present.

Consultant medical staff, frequently excluding junior medical staff or nursing staff, invariably does discussions with family. These staff are often not aware of what has been communicated, which obviously may contribute to subsequent confusion, as the resident medical staff, or rarely, the nurse then does further communication out of routine hours.

The heterogeneity of the population is reflected in the varied reactions of relatives following a completely free and frank discussion. Some profusely thank the intensivist for spending time and finally giving them a clear and pragmatic picture. Others get upset with what they perceive as unnecessary pessimistic statements and later only communicate with the primary consultant. Some families want guarantees regarding the outcome and it falls on the intensivist to explain that all decisions, including withdrawing of life support, will have some degree of uncertainty.

The changing medical paradigm, moving from paternalism to autonomy, also affects doctor–relative communication. This is best illustrated when taking consent for a procedure, for example, a tracheostomy. Few relatives want to know the details of the procedure or the risk involved. In fact, they often cut short the discussion and request that they just sign the form, as in their view, if we feel it is necessary we should just got on with it. Paternalism versus autonomy also functions at a relative–patient level. Patients are unfortunately rarely involved in decisions. Even those clearly conscious, lucid, and communicative are rarely if ever asked to sign a consent form for a procedure or operation. Instead, relatives typically complete these forms, sometimes with a minimal and cursory statement to the patient. This form of obtaining consent is actually legally invalid, but is still widely practiced.

Japan

Satoru Hashimoto

Traditionally in Japan, the disclosure of a moribund condition such as cancer or other terminal condition to the patient is rare compared to Western society, especially when death is imminent. Do not resuscitate orders (DNR) are rare in Far East countries, such as Japan, Korea, and China. So are orders of withdrawal or withholding of aggressive treatment.[1]

Healthcare providers sometimes have to keep the information secret to the dying patient to appease the family's wishes. People who support patient's autonomy are still a minority in Japan because individuality is not viewed in the same way as in the Western countries. In other Far East countries, such as China or Korea, people value harmony within the small blood-related group rather than patient autonomy. However, they also have been influenced by the wave of globalization and their attitude is dramatically changing now.

Advance directives, especially living wills, are now attracting growing interest in Japan although it is not completely accepted yet.[2] Personally, I feel the physician's attitudes are improving with regard to the acceptance of the patient's individual autonomy. About 20 years ago, most cancer patients in Japan did not have a chance to know their real diagnosis, at the behest of their family. Nowadays, most of the patients are informed about their true diagnosis unless death is imminent. Japanese doctors, especially under 50 years old, are less paternalistic and are more willing to discuss end-of-life issues with the patient and the family. But many Japanese view surrogate decision by family as most important for the end-of-life decisions. Also, with national health insurance that covers all Japanese citizens, almost all expenses will be reimbursed. That creates an incentive to insist every expensive therapy be done for unlikely recovery potential. The family does not have to worry about the expensiveness of the therapy in the intensive care unit (ICU).

As it pertains to high-technology critical care, Japan has had very few cadaveric heart or liver transplants (only four hearts and five livers were transplanted in 2004) since the 1997 law allowing organ harvesting after brain death. Diagnosis of brain death is very strict and complex in Japan. Doctors usually prefer to wait for complete cardiac arrest to call death, even if the brain is clearly dead. I have observed many family members, nurses, and doctors look at the heart monitor rather than the dying patient to see the final cardiac beat at the bedside. I even sometimes urge family to express their farewell to the patient and switch off the monitor as soon as possible to avoid dwelling on several more sporadic heartbeats.

It is also interesting to appreciate the general attitude of Japanese people toward religion. The Japanese are more or less influenced by the integrated polytheistic chaos of Shintoism, Buddhism, Confucianism, Taoism, and Catholicism.[3] However, it is very hard to find a hospital that provides a chapel, church, or other religious counterparts. Many Japanese do not profess their belief publicly. Many people mix and match, attending a Shinto shrine 100 days after their birth, wed at the Christian church, and opt for Buddhist funerals. All these factors combine to affect a regional uniqueness in terms of acceptance of death by individuals and their families in Japan, a complex issue for foreigners to understand. Accordingly, I will explain my own views toward ICU end-of-life issues that may not reflect the usual Japanese stereotype.

Full-time clinical intensivists are relatively rare in Japan. In my district, there are over 7000 medical doctors serving a 2.5 million population, and I am one of only 8 full-time intensivists in this area. Five full-time and 15 part-time intensivists work in our hospital with 12 semiclosed ICU beds for 800 general ward beds. The ICU has at least 1:1 nurse/patient ratio for day shifts and 1:2 ratio at night. We only have two medical social workers in the hospital that mainly work for community medicine and have no time to take care of families of dying patients. Thus, only nurses and physicians play a major role dealing with the issue of end of life. The intensivists meet with attending physicians or surgeons every morning and evening and discuss their combined strategy. Usually, during the daytime, intensivists treat ICU patients. The attending surgeons or physicians do their own routine work outside the ICU, but they also deal with the patient's family when they are available.

Intensivist's discussions with family members become more "intense" when the issue of end-of-life care emerges. My role in dealing with end of life frequently begins upon request by the nursing staff. Frequently, I talk to the family members under duress and I try to offer a second expert opinion on outcome under the circumstances. I normally explain the options of withdrawal or withholding life support and explain why this is a humane option, from the vantage of an expert in life support. I explain to the family that current medical procedures may no longer save or improve life but possibly end life or prolong suffering. But I also promise them that we will at least continue to apply "ordinary" care for comfort and relief of suffering. We allow family to meet the patient freely (it is usually limited in the ICU in Japan), and sometimes recommend that the patient be transferred to the comfort ward with mechanical ventilation so the family can continue to be with them during comfort measures.

Some families may refuse to accept my proposal and insist to continue therapy that will prolong suffering. In these cases, we wait, continuing to gently talk with them until they eventually accept their beloved one's inevitable outcome. In Japan, finances and expenses do not enter into patient care at the physician–patient level. Some patients absorb over US $100,000 per month at the end of their life for open-ended aggressive care that simply prolongs death. We have no practical way of dealing with this problem other than by simply waiting and continuing a dialogue with families.

References

1. Levin PD, Sprung CL. Cultural differences at the end of life. Crit Care Med 2003;31(5 Suppl):S354–S357.
2. Masuda Y, Fetters MD, Hattori A, et al. Physicians's reports on the impact of living wills at the end of life in Japan. J Med Ethics 2003;29:248–252.
3. Konishi E. Nurses' attitudes towards developing a do not resuscitate policy in Japan. Nurs Ethics 1998;5:218–227.

2
Critical Illness and End-of-Life Issues: A Global View

An Evaluation of International Medical Ethics at the End of Life

Errington C. Thompson

In the United States, we have had considerable difficulty tackling end-of-life issues in the intensive care unit (ICU). With medicine and pharmacology making more and more advances, bedside clinicians are facing questions that were not asked 20 or 30 years ago. The answers (some, but not all) are somewhat nebulous. For the most part, medical specialists seem unwilling or unable to answer or address these questions. Critical care physicians are uniquely placed to address end-of-life issues. The formula used by most critical care physicians is direct communication with the family in an atmosphere in which family members can interact with the medical team. The critical care physicians use many personnel to help them with this task, including ICU nurses and hospital clergy. It is important for the critical care team to address the family's goals for therapy.

As we turn to investigate how the rest of the world confronts end-of-life issues in the ICU, we will compare and contrast it to the ideal American model. In some parts of the world critical care and end-of-life issues are simply not a problem. This occurs largely in Third World countries. Medical care in these regions of the world is not advanced. Simple first aid maybe the only type of medical care available. Decisions of whether or not to remove a loved one from the ventilator are simply not an issue. These areas are significantly impoverished. Transportation and communication in these areas can also be sparse and inefficient. Economics is the major problem. There are no ICUs. There are no critical care physicians. There are no first responder helicopters or ambulances. In these areas of the world infrastructure needs to be developed in order to support medical clinics, smaller hospitals, and, finally, larger tertiary centers. In these areas medicine must focus on the basics, such as hygiene and clean water.

From India to South Africa, from Buenos Aires to Australia, all of these countries plus many in between have diverse populations of people concentrated in major cities and also have vast territories of open land that may resemble Third World countries. Medical care is highly variable depending upon where you are in the country. In a major city, medical care may resemble that of any major city in United States. On the other hand, in the rural areas, transportation may be difficult. Communication between the rural areas and the major cities may vary from excellent to nonexistent.

In South Africa, human immunodeficiency virus (HIV) and trauma have reached epidemic proportions.[1,2] Therefore, end-of-life medical ethics in many cases has taken a backseat to the practicality of bed space. Physicians in these areas have learned to triage patients who they can help into the ICU and patients that are terminal or preterminal out of the ICU. Patients with severe head injuries do not get long trials of mechanical ventilation. Instead they get 72 hours. After 72 hours, if the patient has not shown significant improvement (Glasgow coma scale <greater than> 10), the patient gets extubated and transferred to the floor. These practices commonly occur at county hospitals (personal communication with R. Eric Hodgson, MD, Nelson R Mandela School of Medicine, Durban, KwaZulu-Natal, South Africa). Interestingly, a county hospital refused renal dialysis for a patient with chronic renal failure. The hospital stated that the patient was not a transplant candidate and therefore had an incurable disease. This decision was challenged in court and was upheld in South Africa.[3] In contrast, at the private hospitals, critical care is delivered much as it is delivered in the United States. These patients have the means to pay for their care. Discussions with the family center on what goals the family would like for the patient. These patients do get tracheostomies and feeding tubes and eventually are transferred to extended care facilities.

Family discussions about goals can take on a different meaning if there are cultural and language barriers. In the United States, greater than 92% of the population speaks English fluently.[4] Another 4% to 4.5% speak Spanish. In Africa, there are a host of languages. Interpreters are frequently needed. Miscommunication occurs quite often, especially when a family member is doing the interpreting (personal communication with R. Eric Hodgson, MD, Nelson R Mandela School of Medicine, Durban, KwaZulu-Natal, South Africa). Family members may interject or delete words or phrases in order to avoid bearing bad news. End-of-life discussions that are already difficult become almost impossible if the physician cannot accurately communicate with the family. Many of these cultures are extremely paternalistic. Therefore, no decision is made without the dominant male figure present. Discussions with other family members are near useless because they will wait for the head of the household or clan to make any decision (personal communication with R. Eric Hodgson, MD, Nelson R Mandela School of Medicine, Durban, Kwa-Zulu-Natal, South Africa).

By contrast, in India, non–critical care specialists deliver the majority of critical care. India has a vast heterogeneous population. There are many cultural, religious, and socioeconomic barriers. Space is a common problem. Having the space to sit down and talk to a family is important in these discussions. Standing out in the hallway is not appropriate. Therefore, many of these discussions are performed under less than ideal circumstances. Because of cultural mores, many family members do not want to hear anything negative that the critical care team has to say. While discussing the risks and benefits of a particular procedure, the family may commonly interrupt the physician and state, "That is fine. Do whatever you think is necessary." It should be reiterated that this practice of not wanting to hear anything negative or bad is not isolated to India but is also seen throughout the world, including the United States. This practice can be frustrating to critical care physicians and nurses who thrive on open dialogue. Open and honest discussions are a cornerstone to informed consent and patient autonomy. Under these circumstances, physicians are forced to do the best they can to communicate everything they can with the family (personal communication with Farhad N. Kapadia, MD, India).

Although I have previously mentioned religion in this chapter, I really have not covered the topic. As we investigate practices in Brazil, religion, specifically Catholicism, looms large. In this Latin American country, the vast majority of citizens are Roman Catholic. Therefore, any discussion of end-of-life issues without including Catholicism would be incomplete. The clergy are an integral part of many critical care teams in Brazil. They play an important part in bridging the gap between the physician and the patient's family. They help with communication. They can help a family understand the patient's grave prognosis. They can also explain that comfort care measures can be and are consistent with Christian teachings. Pope John Paul II in the 1995 encyclical entitled, *The Gospel of Life*,[5] made a distinction between ordinary care and extraordinary care. Extraordinary care is not mandatory and can be burdensome. This would include intubation of a patient who has metastatic lung cancer. Ordinary care, according to Pope John Paul II, would include food or water. This may contradict an earlier 16th century teaching. This topic continues to be an ongoing discussion within the Catholic Church. Critical care providers must be sensitive to these nuances. This is one reason why the clergy should play an integral role to the critical care team not only in Brazil, but also on all critical care teams.

Overcrowding, scarce resources, and insufficient manpower are issues in Brazil as they are all over the world. Triaging ICU beds by moving terminal patients out and more viable patients in is a common practice in Brazil (personal communication with Claudia Teles, MD, Brazil).

There is a commonality as to how critical care providers approach end-of-life issues throughout the world. We all strongly believe in patient autonomy. It would be ideal if all patients had living wills. Unfortunately, this legislation is still evolving in certain parts of the world. In spite of this fact, critical care providers want to know about their patient's wishes. When a patient is incompetent, we turn to the patient's family. It is through the family that the critical care team can get a glimpse at what the patient wishes and believes.

In my communications with physicians throughout the world, I have noticed one dramatic difference in end-of-life issues. In the United States, there are times when patients or their families demand treatment even if it may be futile. This does not seem to be a problem anywhere but in the United States. Australia and England have healthcare systems similar to ours, in which ICU care and critical care providers are widely available. There are two possibilities: either critical care providers in these countries are more amenable to patient demands or patients and patients' families are more likely to accept the critical care team's assessments. This interesting topic will require more investigation.

References

1. Meel BL. Incidence and patterns of violent and/or traumatic deaths between 1993 and 1999 in the Transkei region of South Africa. J Trauma 2004;57:125–129.
2. Heyns Adu P, Benjamin RJ, Swanevelder JP, et al. Prevalence of HIV-1 in blood donations following implementation of a structured blood safety policy in South Africa. JAMA 2006;295:519–526.
3. Thiagraj Soobramoney vs. Minister of Health, Province of Kwazulu-Natal, South Africa. Durban Supreme Court Case Number 5846197, August 1997.
4. Language Use and English-Speaking Ability: 2000. Available at http://www.census. gov/prod/2003pubs/c2kbr-29.pdf. Accessed on February 9, 2006.
5. Pope John Paul II. The gospel of life. Available at: http://www.vatican.va/holy_ father/john_paul_ii/encyclicals/documents/hf_jp-ii_enc_2503199evangelium-vitae_ en.html. Accessed on February 9, 2006.

Communication in the Intensive Care Unit

Richard Burrows

Do not try to live forever – you will not succeed.[1]

The decision to stop treatment and allow death to occur would, prima fascie, appear to be a simple duty of bringing the news to the relatives and allowing them to make the decision to stop in the light of rational medical information that further treatment is unreasonable. It should be clear at the outset that the problem is not in forcing an unwanted operation or treatment onto a patient that all would agree is not only unethical but also illegal. Instead, it is a problem whereby there is an insistence that treatment is continued against advice that the probability of survival is beyond the practicable. This insistence may come either from the relatives, the patient, or the clinician[2] and may be based on a refusal to accept the situation or a failure in communication or both.

Immediately the problem of communication should be manifest as more than the written or spoken word (as can be demonstrated on any football terrace on any given Saturday anywhere in the world!). It necessarily includes undertones of posture, eye contact, hand movement, and so on that would normally be expected to support the spoken word but which may, instead, lead to messages that are interpreted as diametrically opposed to the intended message, ultimately leading to a total loss of trust between all concerned whence the only arbiter is legal action. It is therefore important to understand some of the underlying factors that give rise to nonverbal communication.

Communication involves the use of words that may have very different meanings for some. The distinction between *reasonable* and *rational* carries different meanings although the words are often used interchangeably. Following Rawls,[3] *rational* agents "use the power of judgment and deliberation to seek their own ends," while *reasonable* agents are "ready to propose principles and standards as fair terms of cooperation and to abide by them willingly given the assurance that others will likely do so." Economic arguments are based on judgment and logic[4] that become dangerous when used by politicians to silence debate and are of particular interest in the acquired immunodeficiency syndrome (AIDS) epidemic of South Africa. The same logic may be applied to the resource availability to patients in intensive care as administrators close down on budgets for economic reasons. The only legal challenge to the government in South Africa in respect of "resource allocation" was decided in favor of the government because "resources are limited and choices have to be made."[5] The authorities decide what the resources are but the clinician must make the choices! The upshot is that the clinician's "reasonable" may be so far removed from that of the patient that neither appears to be "rational."

There is the problem of shortfalls in resources and, as a consequence, the allocation of those resources in a manner that is, or is perceived to be, inequitable.[5] That there are shortfalls cannot be questioned — it is only a matter as to where the line is to be drawn. Death occurs in 100% of people and where there is a propensity to throw technology at death in an attempt to forestall that death, this propensity will breed its own shortfall leading to the same arguments. It is difficult to decide what the level of services to the community should be but it seems that the number of beds should be of the order of 6 ICU beds and 11 high-dependency beds/100,000 population.[6] In 1998, the number of public beds in KwaZulu-Natal[7] was 1.25 beds/100,000. Today the number is less than 1 due to closure of hospitals and ICUs. The situation is worse in countries such as Zambia.[8] The disparity between countries such as New Zealand with 5.5 beds/100,000 and South Africa should be instantly apparent. Not so apparent is the disparity between public and private in South Africa, where such disparities can be quickly transformed into debilitating arguments between "haves" and "have nots." Under the circumstances severe rationing has to take place in the public sector and has been addressed in South Africa.[9] But expecting relatives to be reasonable and accept that the bed is to be saved for a patient with a better chance of survival simply does not work, especially if the clinician is in the untenable situation of being seen to be serving a number of masters[10] — the patient or the coffers of society. How does a clinician say to a family that 30 days in ICU has meant that there is now no budget to treat several people with reversible diseases such as tetanus, chest trauma, and eclampsia? Or, on the other hand, other patients have not been admitted while a recalcitrant family exercises their "right" to an ICU bed and the clinician's "right" to test the limits of technology against the inevitability of death — especially in view of the fallibility of prognosis.

Prognosis is an issue of probability where the only certainty is that a clinician will be wrong at some stage. Where there is an imperative of certainty it is not difficult to understand the difficulties clinicians have in bringing such news to a family. To appear to be certain in the face of probabilities or possibilities can easily be communicated as arrogance or overconfidence whereas uncertainty can be read as weakness.

Few clinicians will stand their ground under the pressures likely to befall them under these circumstances.[11] Even if the judgment of the clinician is correct the pressures may be intolerable as demonstrated by the recent Schiavo case. For the clinician under pressure it is far easier to offer treatment with a vanishing chance of success on the basis that at least something is being done. And, in the words of Shaw: "Operation is the safe side as well as the lucrative side for the surgeon."[12] It is what the clinician is paid to do.

Contrary to conventional wisdom, thinking is a process that is aimed at the achievement of a goal[13] that may well be contrary to advice — we see what we want to see and we hear what we want to hear. Perhaps too, we often speak but do not say what we want to say preferring to hide the agenda of our thoughts. We might, unconsciously, be somewhat less than honest believing "honesty to be the best policy" — a policy that Samuel Johnson had little truck with, stating, "The man who believes that honesty is the best policy is not an honest man." A science exists, pseudo and otherwise, that attempts to detect the utterance of an untruth — and it exists side by side with various attempts to beat the polygraph. Although doctors working in ICU can in no way be (usually!) construed as criminals, they may well approach relatives with information they know can be open to question. It is not difficult to understand the reasons why only an individual with a supreme, arrogant belief in his infallibility could approach relatives thus without giving away subliminal messages open to different interpretations.

Then there has been a change in the practice of medicine such that "withdrawal was the proper service a physician rendered to his patient's good death"[14] seems to be no longer acceptable. Illich notes that instruction on how to discriminate between the curable and incurable disappeared from American medical school teaching in 1910. Medicine, according to Illich, has moved from a failure of the doctor/death struggle to a technological systems failure where autonomous individuals should make their own decisions. But at the same time individuals may avoid the necessary difficult problems or decisions in a manner consistent with Dostoyevsky's insight that despite protest, humans do not want freedom or responsibility to make decisions.[15] This is particularly true in respect of advance directives that on face value would appear to go a long way in solving the problem but are characterized by their comparative rarity, which, because death is a frightening issue for most, is hardly surprising that many people refuse to face their own mortality. The situation has been compounded by a legal system, particularly in the United States, that has traditionally viewed medical decisions as paternalistic and unacceptable. At best such a system allows reasonable people to communicate their wishes and find a way forward. At worst it forces an individual, ill-equipped to deal with his own mortality to withdraw within himself, take no further part in the situation, and leave his affairs to be decided on by others who may themselves be unable to communicate on a level acceptable to all concerned.

And there are cultural differences, religious differences, differences of class, political differences, differences of sex, etc., that can also come into the equation and influence the exchange between doctor and patient/relative. It is clear, and should be expected, that the oriental approach will be different from the occidental approach and this is outlined, inter alia, in the manner whereby the female is "protected" from bad news in Japan. In other parts of the world, a similar paternalism exists and is complicated by laws based more on a dogmatic interpretation than in secular argument of justice and fairness — to the point that, on one end of the scale, crime is acceptable to preserve life and on the other end of the scale the outcome is in God's hands. The religious argument removes the problem from human discourse and allows no decision other than that communicated by a Higher Being through His prophet.

Under the circumstances, it should be viewed as surprising that the bulk of communications between doctor and patient/relative takes place in a sense of trust and without any major difficulty but there still remains the occasional situation when, for any one of a variety of reasons, there is a dispute and a refusal to agree to stop. Under the circumstances society weighs heavily with a decision to continue. From the point of view of medical oaths the situation is similar — the imperative is to save life. The flaw in the imperative, where genuine resource issues are concerned, is that no mechanism exists in any oath as to how to choose between patients. It is not uncommon in the public service of South Africa to be asked to take a patient with a likely terminal disease and a few hours later to be asked to admit a patient with eclampsia. Oftentimes too, the communication between the clinicians suffers from a degree of "terminological inexactitude" in order to shift the burden of the problem.

In spite of constant and prolonged communication, conflict may still arise, as in the patient spoken of by Dr. Teles (see Chapter 1), and here in South Africa, just as elsewhere, there is no reasonably agreed rapid mechanism to address the problem of conflict other than waiting for some situation such as a resistant pneumonia to develop wherein treatment is denied as futile (and an ethical fraud!) or going to the courts. In both situations deserving cases are denied treatment and at some point cognizance will have to be given to some form of agreement that a medical decision to stop, arrived at by consensus among experienced healthcare providers, is given legal standing. It is clear that in the United Kingdom at least the pendulum appears to be returning to an approach that places more weight on the fair and just medical decision to stop treatment.

References

1. Shaw GB. Prologues. In: The doctor's dilemma. London: Oldhams Press; 1938:280.
2. Paris JJ. Manslaughter or a legitimate parental decision? The Messenger Case. J Perinatol 1996;16:60–64.
3. Rawls J. Political liberalism. New York: Columbia University Press; 1993:49–50.
4. Nattrass N. The moral economy of AIDS in South Africa. Cambridge: Cambridge University Press; 2004:35–40.
5. Hardin G. The tragedy of the commons. Science 1968;162:1243–1248.
6. Lyons RA, Wareham K, Hutchings HA, Major E, Fergusen B. Population requirement for adult critical care beds: a prospective, quantitative and qualitative study. Lancet 2000;335:595–598.
7. Bhagwanjee S. Audit of intensive care utilisation in Kwazulu-Natal.
8. Watters D. Intensive care in Zambia. Intensive Care World 1989;6:211–215.
9. Thiagraj Soobramoney vs. Minister of Health, Province of Kwazulu-Natal, South Africa. Durban Supreme Court Case Number 5846197, August 1997.
10. Levinsky NG. The doctors master. N Engl J Med 1984;311:1573–1575.
11. Dyer C. London hospital to face high court for allegedly refusing to resuscitate disabled girl. BMJ 2004;328:125.
12. Shaw GB. Prologues. In: The doctor's dilemma. London: Oldhams Press; 1938.
13. Dörner D. The logic of failure. New York: Basic Books; 1996:17.
14. Illich I. Death undefeated: from mediclisation to systematisation. BMJ 1995;311:1652–1653.
15. Paris JJ, Muir JC, Reardon FE. Ethical and legal issues in intensive care. J Intensive Care Med 1977;12:298–309.

End-of-Life Issues in the Critically Ill: A Global Perspective

Donald B. Chalfin

Critical care delivery differs significantly from nation to nation across the world in terms of such fundamental aspects as physician oversight and intensivist supervision, nurse-to-patient ratios, patient triage, admission and discharge criteria, the presence of other healthcare professionals such as respiratory therapists and pharmacologists, available technology, and the number of allowable intensive care unit (ICU) beds. From the standpoint of critical care organization and ICU structure, certain healthcare systems, such as Australia and New Zealand, have strict and uniform standards and mandates regarding intensivist responsibilities and the number of nurses required to staff a unit whereas others — most notably the United States — are characterized by wide variability in unit structure, critical care organization, and intensivist availability.[1-3] In addition, there is also wide variability among (and even within) nations in patient-specific characteristics such as case mix, severity of illness, and primary diagnosis. While some of this variation may depend upon the availability of ICU beds (relative to the number of other acute care beds) along with the presence of viable alternatives such as step-down and intermediate care units and even skilled nursing facilities that can properly care for ventilated patients, much of it can be attributed to community-, region-, and nation-specific cross-cultural factors ranging from religious differences, unique demographic features, and different societal expectations.

Despite these and other differences, there are certain unifying factors of critical care delivery that are common to all healthcare systems across the world. While the cost of health care and its percentage of gross domestic product (GDP) for individual nations may differ considerably throughout the world, one can safely say that critical care nevertheless consumes a disproportionate share of every nation's inpatient and overall healthcare expenditures. Furthermore, one can make the case that ICUs share a certain "generic commonality" and overall intuitive "gestalt," to the point that a healthcare provider from one nation would likely recognize another nation's ICU without much, if any, difficulty. Finally and perhaps most importantly, an overall clinical convergence has emerged regarding the recognition of certain societal imperatives and fundamental patient rights that transcend cultural and national boundaries, rights that become especially important with respect to end-of-life issues and the provision of care to those for whom death is imminent.

In all cultures, intensivists and other physicians, ICU nurses, and other healthcare professionals are increasingly called upon to provide end-of-life and related palliative care. This often presents a conflict to the physician, in the sense that it challenges the seemingly paramount tenet (and perhaps even the physician's ego) to provide and search for a cure and instead focus primarily on the alleviation of pain and the provision of comfort. Perhaps in certain cultures, this conflict becomes more manifest than in others, as evident by international differences in physicians' attitudes towards end of life, which manifest by different approaches to the decision to initiate and the propensity to withdraw care in a critically ill patient.[4] These differences go beyond the mere attitudes and beliefs of the healthcare provider and actually become evident in such practical aspects of end-of-life care as the timing of withdrawal of care, the method and mode of communication of preferences, prognoses, and treatment options to patients and their families, and the retention and delineation of decisionmaking powers. Furthermore, international differences also show up in the decision to even refer and potentially admit a patient to the ICU versus the provision of care in a less aggressive (and less expensive) setting.[5] While the attitudes and practice patterns of physicians and other healthcare providers greatly influence the care that is provided at the end of life, one needs to remain cognizant that patient and societal mores and beliefs are also key determinants in the provision of end-of-life and palliative care. Certain societies and cultures, for example, place great value on patient autonomy and complete disclosure of all information, whereas other cultures attempt to "protect" and "shield" a patient from bad news and even participation in their own therapeutic decisions.

Medical care may be viewed as a reflection of a nation's and a society's core values and guiding priorities, not only for the care that is provided to an individual patient but also with respect to overall public health measures and goals. This notion is perhaps increasingly evident with respect to end-of-life issues and the provision of palliative care and comfort and supportive measures. Clearly then, cultural and national mores and constraints play a key role in determining how, where, and what care and support is delivered and the overall approach to end-of-life care and thus, providers in all societies must be attuned to a patient's particular value set and cultural makeup. While these international and cross-cultural differences are likely to impede efforts to create international standards and guidelines for end-of-life care in the critically ill, one can certainly argue that palliative and end-of-life care must become an integral part of any ICU service across the world.

References

1. Australian College of Critical Care Nurses. Position statement on intensive care nursing staffing. Aust Crit Care 2002;15:6–7.
2. Venkatesh B, Kruger P, Pascoe RL, Morgan TJ. Intensive care in Australia and New Zealand: past, present and future. Natl Med J India 2004;17:107–108.
3. Pronovost PJ, Angus DC, Dorman T. Physician staffing patterns and clinical outcomes in critically ill patients: a systematic review. JAMA 2002;288:2151–2162.
4. Yaguchi A, Truog RD, Curtis JR, et al. International differences in end-of-life attitudes in the intensive care unit. Arch Intern Med 2005;165:1970–1975.

5. Carlet J, Thijs LF, Antonelli M, et al. Challenges in end-of-life care in the ICU: statement of the 5th Intenrational Consensus Conference in Critical Care. Brussels, Belgium. April 2003. Intensive Care Med 2004;30:770–784.

3
Death in a Lonely Place: Pathophysiology of the Dying Patient

Mike Darwin and Phil Hopkins

> He is miserable, that dieth not before he desires to die.
>
> —Thomas Fuller

In the long arc that is my memory I cannot forget her. It was over 20 years ago and that is in good measure the tragedy of this tale; that with the passing of an entire human generation her story is still current, still common, still haunting the corridors of critical care medicine. It was just another day starting at 0600 hours as they all did then. My first patient was a new admission to ICU. The first line in the chart's most recent entry elicited an involuntary groan. This 24-year-old African–American female was admitted to the ICU at 0200 with multisystem organ failure secondary to *E. coli* septicemia following an intrauterine death. The narrative that followed described a patient in extremis with refractory septic shock, diffuse intravascular coagulation, and adult respiratory distress syndrome, a woman who was clearly dying. As I primed the dialysis circuit with salt-poor albumin I recoiled as I glimpsed a photograph left by her distraught husband. It showed a beautiful, smiling, vibrant woman with extraordinary violet eyes. How had she gone from this to near death in the ICU in just over 24 hours?

Since this case occurred, stellar advances have been made in our understanding of the human response to microbial challenge. Until recently, the focus was on downstream pro-inflammatory immunology. However, in the last decade an insight has been gained into the sophisticated biological processes that occur at the host–pathogen interface. In particular, we have begun to understand how the host first senses invading pathogens and how this recognition is signaled to the innate and adaptive immune systems.

The Recognition of Infection

The Pattern Recognition of Microbe-Associated Molecular Patterns

In recent years, a detailed understanding of the host–pathogen interface has been developed. It is now clear that the mammalian host has a genetically encoded memory for a highly restricted number of conserved component structures and toxins from invading pathogens.[1,2] Host interaction with these microbe-associated molecular patterns (MAMPs) can lead to either inflammation (or disease) or to the establishment of a mutually beneficial eukaryotic–prokaryotic association.[3,4] Here we use pattern recognition of Gram-negative organisms to illustrate the sophisticated biology underlying this process.

Pattern Recognition of Gram-Negative Microbes

Lipopolysaccharide (LPS) is the dominant MAMP in the pattern recognition of Gram-negative bacteria. LPS alone is sufficient to induce shock and many of the other systemic host responses seen in sepsis when given experimentally to laboratory animals or human volunteers.[5,6] In one study of the 488 genes upregulated by whole cell *Escherichia coli*, 88% of the gene transcript profile was replicated on exposure to purified LPS alone.[7] The markedly reduced pro-inflammatory potential of a lipid A–deficient strain of *Neisseria meningitides* has further revealed the dominant role of LPS.[8] Finally, LPS is released into serum containing Gram-negative microbes in vitro and into the circulation of critically ill patients.[9–11] There are multiple sources for LPS within the circulation of such individuals. These include direct infection, inoculation from intravascular devices, and translocation from injured organs such as ventilated lungs and the gastrointestinal tract.[12,13] The use of antibiotics may further increase levels of circulating LPS.[14]

Lipopolysaccharide-Binding Proteins and Pattern-Recognition Receptors

The biological activity of LPS, as the dominant MAMP in the pathogenesis of Gram-negative sepsis, is mediated by a complex system of soluble binding proteins, cell surface receptors, and intracellular pattern-recognition structures. Many (such as LBP and CD14) have been cloned and studied in detail. This pattern-recognition system is coupled with sophisticated intracellular signaling pathways that lead to induction of transcriptional controls for inflammatory gene expression.

After its release from Gram-negative bacteria, there is binding competition for LPS from LPS-binding protein (LBP) and high-density lipoprotein (HDL). LPS bound to LBP is then transferred to soluble or membrane-associated CD14.[15,16] Membrane-associated CD14 is not only a functional receptor for LPS: it also has a biologically distinct scavenging role.[17] The functional role of CD14 is also limited by the absence of any intracellular signaling apparatus. Instead, a member of the interleukin 1 receptorlike family, toll-like receptor (TLR) 4, constitutes the dominant transmembrane pattern recognition system for LPS, facilitating sophisticated pro-inflammatory signal transduction. The discovery of TLR4 was based on the observation that the LPS-resistant C3H/Hej and C57BL/10ScCr mice have a mutation and complete deletion of the *tlr4* gene, respectively.[18] In addition, TLR4 knockout mice do not respond to LPS.[19] Finally, transfection of TLR4 into LPS unresponsive cell lines can restore LPS responses.[20] Importantly, each LPS pattern-recognition receptor should not be viewed in isolation. Instead, they are now known to form a dynamic multimeric receptor complex within the lipid raft.[21] Indeed, an additional adapter protein, MD2, is also known to play an important role in CD14-TLR4 LPS pattern recognition.[22] A more detailed understanding of events following LPS pattern recognition at this multimeric complex has recently been obtained.[23] The signal transduction process following pattern recognition of LPS is highly complex.[24] A number of other cell surface (CD11b/CD18, RP105) and intracellular receptors (NOD1/2) are also known to be capable of LPS pattern recognition, although their relevance in vivo is uncertain.[21,25,26]

Although it was not the first TLR to be cloned, the discovery of TLR4, and a subsequent investigation of its biology, provided a platform for the discovery and investigation of 10 other human TLRs, each with the capacity for specific and distinct pattern-recognition properties.[27] Not only does pattern recognition trigger immediate innate immune responses, but it also directs subsequent adaptive immunity primarily through the designation and targeted differentiation of dendritic cells.[28] Beutler has suggested that the narrow target or "hourglass" immunological profile offered by the pattern-recognition process makes it a natural target for adjuvant immune interventions.[29]

The Response to Infection

Antimicrobial Peptides and the Activation of Complement

The release of antimicrobial peptides such as lysozyme, β-defensins, cathelicidins, and bactericidal permeability–increasing protein at epithelial surfaces and within the intravascular compartment provides the most immediate response to potential injurious invasion from pathogenic microbes.[30,31] The amphipathic, hydrophobic, and cationic peptides operate through microbial membrane depolarization and cell wall lytic enzyme activation.[32,33] They are constitutively expressed to prevent colonization or biofilm formation, and upregulated via defined signal transduction pathways in active infection.[34,35] Cecropin peptides have also been shown to be as efficacious as conventional antibiotics in the therapy of septic shock in animal models.[36]

The three complement cascades (classical, alternative, and mannose-binding lectin pathways) are also pivotal in the innate response to microbial challenge.[37] Complement is activated on bacterial surfaces and by bacterial products such as LPS, acute-phase proteins (e.g., C-reactive protein), and immune complexes. This leads to enhanced opsonization and direct lysis of invading organisms through the assembly of the terminal attack complex C5b-9. In addition, release of the anaphylotoxins C3a and C5a exert a number of proinflammatory effects, such as promoting chemotactic responses of neutrophils, augmentation of superoxide anion production, vasodilatation, and increased vascular permeability.[38–40] However, complement activation is a double-edged sword. Complement has been shown to suppress neutrophil-mediated innate immunity and elevated levels of C5a in septic patients have been associated with reduced survival.[41,42] Indeed, blockade of C5a has had beneficial effects in an experimental sepsis models.[43,44]

Acute Activation of the Endothelium and Coagulation Cascade

The endothelium plays a dominant role in the host response to sepsis. It facilitates targeted immune cell margination and extravasation (through expression of adhesion molecules and release of cytokines and chemokines); releases nitric oxide to modulate vascular tone; and regulates coagulation and fibrinolysis.[45–47] A detailed review of endothelial responses is beyond the remit of this chapter. However, it is worth noting that endothelial responses exhibit the same double-edged nature as other immune responses in the context of sepsis. Although nitric oxide (NO) release and upregulation of adhesion molecules (e.g., lymphocyte function associated antigen 1; intercellular adhesion molecule 1; endothelial leucocyte adhesion molecule 1; L-selectin, and P-selectin) are involved in proinflammatory tissue damage, blockade of these factors can have adverse effects in septic shock.[48,49]

The septic endothelium provokes injurious thrombin generation and fibrin deposition through the release of tissue factor and platelet activating factor. This underpins the general and profound dysregulation of the normal human coagulation response observed in severe sepsis.[50,51] There is evidence of consumption of platelets and coagulation factors such as factor VII leading to disseminated intravascular coagulation in some cases. Depressed levels of endogenous inhibitors of coagulation such as protein C and antithrombin III also reflect the severity of the septic insult.[52–54] Notably, the augmentation of systemic protein C concentrations provides the only successful adjuvant therapy in sepsis to date.[55–57]

Activation of Immune Cells

Neutrophils, lymphocytes, and monocytes all exhibit specific activation characteristics in sepsis. Neutrophil-mediated antimicrobial mechanisms consist of phagocytosis and release of both oxygen-dependent (reactive oxygen species) and oxygen-independent (lactoferrin, azurophil granule enzymes) mediators.[58] Sepsis is associated with the migration of activated neutrophils from the bloodstream into inflamed tissues in parallel with intensive production of more immature cells by the bone marrow. This massive neutrophil flux may account for reports of neutropenia and neutrophil dysfunction in sepsis.[59,60] Although such neutrophils have enhanced respiratory burst activity they are conversely less able to respond to further stimulation. Neutrophil survival is also prolonged in sepsis due to a reduced constitutive apoptosis rate. Neutrophils are thought to play a key role in the pathogenesis of adult respiratory distress syndrome through massive sequestration within the pulmonary microvasculature and damaging release of oxidants and proteases.[61-63]

In human sepsis there appears to be a subset of monocytes responsible for the bulk of the proinflammatory response and cytokine production.[64-66] However, this response appears to be limited over time with the development of reduced responsiveness to stimulation with lipopolysaccharide in conjunction with the reduced expression of surface human leuojocyte antigen (IILA)-DR.[67,68] Circulating monocytes also have the capacity to differentiate into tissue macrophages or dendritic cells following migration into tissues across the endothelium. These may be constitutive resident macrophages (such as hepatic Kupffer cells), exhibiting marked heterogeneity according to their microenvoronment.[69] However, a specific subset (CX3CR1 low, CCR2+, CD62L+) are recruited by chemokines (CCL2 and CXCL9) across the activated endothelium (see above) at inflamed tissues.[47,66] Inflammatory macrophages have important phagocytic properties, facilitated through surface complement and Fcγ receptors.

B and T lymphocytes are thought to play a predominant role in adaptive immune responses following antigen recognition by surface immunoglobulin receptors and presentation by major histocompatability complex (MHC) molecules, respectively. The complex interplay that occurs between B and T cells during infection in mammals has been the subject of recent review.[70] During sepsis there is a selective depletion of CD4+ and B lymphocytes by selective apoptosis.[71] This produces a reversal in CD4+/CD8+ ratio and an increase in the release of T helper-2 cytokines (IL-4 and IL-10).71–73 In addition, T cells become relatively anergic, with reduced CD3 expression and lower numbers the γ-δ cell receptor subset.[72-74] In some sepsis models the prevention of lymphocyte apoptosis may improve outcome,[75] while the adoptive transfer of apoptotic splenocytes can worsen prognosis.[76] Another study found that caspase inhibitors, blockers of apoptosis enzyme pathways, are an effective therapy in pneumonia-induced sepsis.[77]

Role of Cytokines and Chemokines

There is good evidence to suggest that cytokines such as tumor necrosis factor α (TNF-α) play a key role in the pathogenesis of severe sepsis. This has been reproducibly demonstrated in vitro and in vivo.[78,79] They operate by induction of synthesis of phospholipase A2 and cyclooxygenase which facilitate the production of eicosanoids and platelet activating factor.[80] Through activation of specific G-protein–coupled receptors these mediators alter vasomotor tone and increase blood flow and vascular permeability. Importantly, the blockade of these cytokines has provided a successful strategy in some models of sepsis.[81-83] Novel cytokine targets, such as macrophage inhibitory factor (MIF) and high mobility group protein B1 (HMGB1), have recently been described.[84-86] Both have direct actions on proinflammatory gene expression.

Chemokines, including IP-10, IL-8, macrophage inflammatory protein (MIP)-1, MIP-2, RANTES, and MCP-1, have an essential role in host defense, controlling the recruitment and activation of immune cells in response to inflammatory stimuli.[87] As with cytokines, conflicting results have been produced by investigators trying to correlate serum chemokine levels with sepsis severity.[88] Patients with septic shock appear to have defective IL-8–mediated neutrophil chemotaxis.[89,90]

The next day, I stared at the white board: her name was still there. Hours turned to days, and days turned to weeks. The wall space around the head of her bed soon became covered with cards and placards with long, handwritten prayers and appeals to God for her recovery. She suffered multiple nosocomial infections and had almost died following hemorrhage after a percutaneous tracheostomy. Her edematous sacrum broke down and became infected with multiresistant microbes. Her abdominal wound became infected with the same organisms and then dehisced, exposing her innards. She suffered recurrent episodes of candidemia and aspergillus was isolated from a cavitating lung lesion. Her bone marrow became aplastic, and she required constant hematological support in the form of platelet and packed red cell infusions. More than once her minister administered some final prayers. She was moved into an isolation room, a transfer justified by her multiresistant infections, but which took the smell of her wounds away from the other patients. Nurses would refuse to spend whole shifts in her room. The worst thing of all was her mouthed plea, in moments of lucidity, to be allowed to die.

The literature surrounding the pathogenesis and therapy of severe human sepsis has almost exclusively concentrated on the early innate response to infection and initial phase of resuscitation. Indeed, attempts to augment conventional antibiotic therapy have focused on the blunting of primary proinflammatory innate responses, deemed to be injurious to the host. There has been a specific concentration on the rapid initial resuscitation (or even preemptive optimization) of such patients.[91,92] However, such studies always identify a population of patients who do not respond and who have a correspondingly dire prognosis.[93] Aggressive correction of oxygen delivery in such patients has resulted in increased mortality.[94,95] Our inability to reverse the dying process in a significant proportion of the patients we inherit is reflected in a number of paradoxical observations which we will now outline.

Paradoxes in Pattern Recognition of Invading Pathogens

While it seems undisputable that LPS constitutes a key microbial component in the etiology of severe Gram-negative sepsis, a complete understanding of its biology, particularly in the context of human critical illness, has not yet been achieved. This is reflected by two unexplained observations in the clinical setting.

1. The absolute level of plasma LPS in patients with severe sepsis does not appear predictive of fever, severity, or outcome, particularly in the absence

of bacteremia.[96–100] This has been confirmed by meta-analysis.[101] Indeed, most patients with endotoxemia and septic shock have low concentrations (<less than> 500 pg/mL). In addition, in some studies LPS levels have not even predicted the presence of Gram-negative bacteremia.[99] For example, many patients with fungal or Gram-positive sepsis have detectable LPS in their bloodstreams. This paradox has also been noted in several animal models. One group has consistently found that Gram-negative organisms most associated with induction of shock produced the lowest levels of endotoxemia.[102,103] In others there was no correlation between the degree of organ injury and levels of systemic endotoxin.[98,104,105]

2. Attempts to block LPS using peptides or antibodies (polyclonal and monoclonal) have failed to reduce mortality in clinical trials.[106–111] In addition, other Gram-negative structures have also been targeted with little success.[112]

A number of explanations for these unexpected observations have been suggested. Firstly, LPS-induced gene expression may be too complex to predict the effects of modulation in complex systems. A recent study using serial analysis of gene expression (SAGE) has revealed the complexity of LPS-induced gene expression in monocytes.[113] Douglas Golenbock's group has demonstrated the potential for further complexity by showing that in mice the majority of this genetic activity is MyD88 independent.[114] Second, experimental systems utilizing pure LPS challenge are now known to poorly replicate the conditions found in clinical sepsis.[115,116] In particular, although disruption of LPS pattern recognition with antibodies, blocking peptides, or genetic manipulation prevents LPS-mediated host injury, this does not occur in models involving bacterial challenge or clinical sepsis. For example, while disruption of the LPS–LBP or LPS–CD14 interaction in mice by antibodies or genetic manipulation reduces LPS-induced lethality, it increases susceptibility to bacterial challenge.[117–124] This may also explain the contrasting success of blockade of simple LPS recognition in humans with the failure of this strategy in the clinical setting.[6,125,126] The hypothesis that such innate immunity plays a crucial role in microbial clearance is supported by some further recent observations, revealing the absolute requirement for intact pattern recognition.[127–130] Importantly, this thesis may also underpin the general failure of any adjuvant therapy (such as anti-TNF agents) designed to blunt inflammatory responses in such patients.

Paradoxes in the Immune Response

We have described the chemical and cellular response to infective challenge. However, it has proved surprisingly difficult to utilize this information to provide either predictive information regarding severity, or strategies for therapy. This is most clearly illustrated by a number of paradoxical observations regarding proinflammatory cytokines.

1. The absolute plasma level of any given cytokine has not proved useful either as an indicator of severity or outcome. While some authors have claimed such an association, attempts to reliably reproduce such observations have failed.[131–137] Meta-analyses of such studies or attempts to use cytokine concentrations in ratios have failed to resolve this problem.[138–142] It is also worth noting that in the clinical setting (with the exception of meningococcal sepsis) that TNF-α levels are actually often very low. Likewise, in sophisticated sepsis models (such as murine caecal ligation puncture) cytokine levels are often considerable lower than those observed in many early studies which utilized infusions of Gram-negative lipopolysaccharides.[131,143–145]

2. An attempt to associate individual cytokine polymorphisms with severity or outcome have produced equally heterogeneous results.[146,147]

3. Finally, and most damaging, multiple attempts to block cytokines as a therapeutic strategy have universally failed.[148–151] The same problem has been replicated with new cytokine targets such as HMGB1 and with other innate immune targets such as platelet activating factor, antithrombin III, tissue factor pathway inhibitor, and nitric oxide.[152–155]

Each day I would come in praying that I would not see her name on the whiteboard with my name next to it. And each day both were there. She moved from near death crisis to near death crisis with her vitals often hovering at levels that we all knew were not survivable — yet she survived. Analgesia was difficult due to hemodynamic instability. Her liver failed, she developed an irreversible metabolic acidosis, and renal replacement therapy became unviable as her cardiac output fell. Mottled and bleeding, she slowly died. She was alone at the end, a nurse summoned to her bed in the night by an alarm. Her death had taken 2 months and 4 days.

Future Hopes and Final Thoughts

Some patients with a critical illness do not respond to initial resuscitation. Instead they enter a phase of protracted multiorgan failure. The pathophysiology of such individuals has not been the subject of detailed investigation. It is clear that host immunity in such patients has been devastated. This profound immunosuppression appears to be precipitated by normal homeostatic control mechanisms such as induction of IL-10 in conjunction with complex leukocyte reprogramming involving the induction of tolerance, the downregulation of HLA-DR, and the control of apoptosis.[72,156,157] The reason for the prolongation of such effects, and the subsequent chronic and cumulative host injury that ensues, is only just being addressed.[158–160] Importantly, not only do such patients have shattered immune systems — they also suffer recurrent and cumulative microbial and iatrogenic injury. The latter includes injurious mechanical ventilation and drug-induced cerebral, liver, and renal injury. However, all these problems are dwarfed by the psychological cost to patients and their relatives as explored by other authors in this publication.

Several approaches have been suggested in such patients. First, there may need to be a change in the use of established conventional therapies such as antibiotics. While there is no doubt that such agents play a key role in the management of sepsis, they cannot be used with impunity.[161–164] They disrupt commensal microflora, encouraging the acquisition of multiresistant nosocomial organisms, exacerbate loss of gut barrier function, and lead to the release of toxic microbial products.[165–168] The double-edged sword of antibiotic therapy has been reflected in the recent debate surrounding the use of selective gut decontamination. While several randomized, controlled clinical trials have shown that this approach can be efficacious in reducing nosocomial infections such as ventilator-associated pneumonia, many investigators have pointed to inherent dangers in such a strategy.[169–171]

Other investigators have suggested that it may be appropriate under some circumstances to boost rather than block host immunity during an episode of severe sepsis. The reconstitution of the immune system has been attempted using cytokines and immune cells.[172–175] However, the timing of such interventions is clearly crucial and the strategy remains unproven in the clinical setting. The potential difficulties are illustrated by attempts to modulate the activity of γ interferon in experimental sepsis models; both inhibition and addition of this lymphokine have been shown to be therapeutic.[176–178] Interestingly, reconstitutive therapy has received support from the only evidence based advances in critical care in the management of severe sepsis. First, there is growing evidence to support compensation for the dysregulated endocrine function and nutritional deficiency seen in these individuals. These include tight control of blood glucose (with insulin); the use of low-dose steroids; the use of low-dose vasopressin, and the augmentation of standard feeding regimes with glutamine and selenium.[179–183] Second, the infusion of protein C, replacing a well-documented deficit, has proved to be the only successful adjuvant therapy in patients with severe sepsis.[55–57]

Despite huge scientific advances, we are still decades from a complete understanding of the biology underpinning the human systemic inflammatory response. In the ICU we often inherit patients who nature intended to die. Unfortunately, to the profound detriment of many of our patients, we still have only partial knowledge; we cannot restore life, only prolong death. Worse still, a lack of reliable physiological and biological predictors prevents us knowing, at the outset of an episode of critical illness, who will live and who will die. We have to fall back on our instincts and humanity. As other authors in this publication have described, we often fail in this respect. Lack of knowledge concerning the systemic inflammatory response is not a failing. However, lack of humanity in the face of a dying patient who is receiving futile supportive care is unforgivable. In the face of partial knowledge, we still need to learn that sometimes it is necessary to replace life-sustaining cold technology with human words and actions to comfort the dying patient. Death is a lonely business; but it need not happen in a lonely place.

References

1. Janeway CA Jr. Approaching the asymptote? Evolution and revolution in immunology. Cold Spring Harb Symp Quant Biol 1990;54:1–13.
2. Matzinger P. Tolerance, danger, and the extended family. Annu Rev Immunol 1994;12:991–1045.
3. Koropatnick TA, Engle JT, Apicella MA, Stabb EV, Goldman WE, McFall-Ngai MJ. Microbial factor-mediated development in a host-bacterial mutualism. Science 2004;306:1186–1188.
4. Rakoff-Nahoum S, Paglino J, Eslami-Varzaneh F, Edberg S, Medzhitov R. Recognition of commensal microflora by toll-like receptors is required for intestinal homeostasis. Cell 2004;118;229–241.
5. DaSilva AMT, Kaulbach HC, Chuidian FS, Lambert DR, Suffredini AF, Danner L. Shock and multiple organ dysfunction after self administration of Salmonella endotoxin. N Engl J Med 1993;328:1457–1460.
6. Bunnell E, Lynn M, Habet K, et al. A lipid A analog, E5531, blocks the endotoxin response in human volunteers with experimental endotoxemia. Crit Care Med 2000;28:2713–2720.
7. Huang Q, Liu D, Majewski P, et al. The plasticity of dendritic cell responses to pathogens and their components. Science 2001;294:870–875.
8. Pridmore AC, Wyllie DH, Abdillahi F, et al. A lipopolysaccharide-deficient mutant of Neisseria meningitidis elicits attenuated cytokine release by human macrophages and signals via toll-like receptor (TLR) 2 but not via TLR4/MD2. J Infect Dis 2001;183:89–96.
9. Levin J, Poore TE, Zauber NP, Oser RS. Detection of endotoxin in the blood of patients with sepsis due to Gram-negative bacteria. N Engl J Med 1970;283:1313–1316.
10. Tesh VL, Duncan RL Jr, Morrison DC. The interaction of Escherichia coli with normal human serum: the kinetics of serum-mediated lipopolysaccharide release and its dissociation from bacterial killing. J Immunol 1986;137:1329–1335.
11. Danner RL, Elin RJ, Hosseini JM, Wesley RA, Reilly JM, Parillo JE. Endotoxaemia in human septic shock. Chest 1991;99:169–175.
12. Haglund U. Systemic mediators released from the gut in critical illness. Crit Care Med 1993;21:S15–S18.
13. Murphy DB, Cregg N, Tremblay L, et al. Adverse ventilatory strategy causes pulmonary-to-systemic translocation of endotoxin. Am J Respir Crit Care Med 2000;162:27–33.
14. Maskin B, Fontan PA, Spinedi EG, Gammella D, Badolati A. Evaluation of endotoxin release and cytokine production induced by antibiotics in patients with Gram-negative nosocomial pneumonia. Crit Care Med 2002;30:349–354.
15. Schumann RR, Leong SR, Flaggs GW, et al. Structure and function of lipopolysaccharide binding protein. Science 1990;249:1429–1431.
16. Wright SD, Ramos RA, Tobias PS, et al. CD14, a receptor for complexes of lipopolysaccharide (LPS) and LPS binding protein. Science 1990;249:1431–1433.
17. Gegner JA, Ulevitch RJ, Tobias PS. Lipopolysaccharide (LPS) signal transduction and clearance. Dual roles for LPS binding protein and membrane CD14. J Biol Chem 1995;270:5320–5325.

18. Poltorak A, He X, Smirnova I, et al. Defective LPS signaling in C3H/HeJ and C57BL/10ScCr mice; mutations in tlr4 gene. Science 1999;282:2085–2088.
19. Takeuchi O, Hoshino K, Kawai T, et al. Differential roles of TLR2 and TLR4 in recognition of Gram-negative and Gram-positive bacterial cell wall components. Immunity 1999;11:443–451.
20. Chow JC, Young DW, Golenbock DT, Crist WJ, Gusovsky F. Toll-like receptor 4 mediates lipopolysaccharide-induced signal transduction. J Biol Chem 1999;274:19689–19692.
21. Triantafilou K, Triantafilou M, Dedrick RL. A CD14-independent LPS receptor cluster. Nat Immunol 2001;2:338–345.
22. Shimazu R, Akashi S, Ogata H, et al. MD-2, a molecule that confers lipopo lysaccharide responsiveness on Toll-like receptor 4. J Exp Med 1999;189:1777–1782.
23. Latz E, Visintin A, Lien E, et al. Lipopolysaccharide Rapidly traffics to and from the Golgi apparatus with the toll-like receptor 4-MD2-CD14 complex in a process that is distinct from the initiation of signal transduction. J Biol Chem 2002;277:47834–47843.
24. Akira S, Takeda K. Toll-like receptor signaling. Nat Rev Immunol 2004;4:499–511.
25. Ingalls RR, Golenbock DT. CD11c/CD18, a transmembrane signaling receptor for lipopolysaccharide. J Exp Med 1995;181:1473–1479.
26. Inohara N, Ogura Y, Chen FF, Muto A, Nunez G. Human Nod1 confers responsiveness to bacterial lipopolysaccharides. J Biol Chem 2001;276:2551–2554.
27. Hopkins P, Sriskandan S. Mammalian toll-like receptors: to immunity and beyond. Clin Exp Immunol 2005;140:395–407.
28. Iwasaki A, Medzhitov R. Toll-like receptor control of the adaptive immune responses. Nat Immunol 2004;5:987–995.
29. Beutler B. Inferences, questions and possibilities in Toll-like receptor signalling. Nature 2004;430:257–263.
30. Fleming A. Lysozyme. Proc R Soc London B Biol Sci 1922;93:306–317.
31. Canny G, Levy O, Furuta GT, et al. Lipid mediator-induced expression of bactericidal/ permeability-increasing protein (BPI) in human mucosal epithelia. Proc Natl Acad Sci U S A. 2002;99:3902–3907.
32. Lee JY, Boman A, Chuanxin S, et al. Antibacterial peptides from pig intestine: isolation of a mammalian cecropin. Proc Natl Acad Sci U S A 1989;86:9159–9162.
33. Zasloff M. Antimicrobial peptides of multicellular organisms. Nature 2002;415:389–395.
34. Singh PK, Parsek MR, Greenberg EP, Welsh MJ. A component of innate immunity prevents bacterial biofilm development. Nature 2002;417:552–554.
35. Kaiser V, Diamond G. Expression of mammalian defensin genes. J Leukoc Biol 2000;68:779–784.
36. Giacometti A, Cirioni O, Ghiselli R, et al. Effect of mono-dose intraperitoneal cecropins in experimental septic shock. Crit Care Med 2001;29:1666–1669.
37. Walport MJ. Complement. New Engl J Med 2001;344:1058–1066.
38. Shin HS, Snyderman R, Friedman E, et al. Chemotactic and anaphylatoxic fragment cleaved from the fifth component of guinea pig complement. Science 1968;162:361–363.
39. Goldstein IM, Weissmann G. Generation of C5-derived lysosomal enzyme-releasing activity (C5a) by lysates of leukocyte lysosomes. J Immunol 1974;113:1583–1588.

40. Sacks T, Moldow CF, Craddock PR, Bowers TK, Jacob HS. Oxygen radicals mediate endothelial cell damage by complement-stimulated granulocytes. An in vitro model of immune vascular damage. J Clin Invest 1978;61:1161–1167.
41. Huber-Lang MS, et al. Complement-induced impairment of innate immunity during sepsis. J Immunol 2002;169:3223–3231.
42. Riedemann NC. Increased C5a receptor expression in sepsis. J Clin Invest 2002;110: 101–108.
43. Stevens JH, et al. Effects of anti-C5a antibodies on the adult respiratory distress syndrome in septic primates. J Clin Invest 1986;77:1812–1816.
44. Czermak BJ, et al. Protective effects of C5a blockade in sepsis. Nat Med 1999;5: 788–792.
45. Palmer RMJ, Ferrige AG, Moncada S. Nitric oxide release accounts for the biological activity of endothelium-derived relaxing factor. Nature 1987;327: 524–526.
46. Annane D, Sanquer S, Sebille V, et al. Compartmentalised inducible nitric-oxide synthase activity in septic shock. Lancet 2000;355:1143–1148.
47. Imhof BA, Aurrand-Lions M. Adhesion mechanisms regulating the migration of monocytes. Nat Rev Immunol 2004;4:432–444.
48. Eichacker PQ, Hoffman WD, Farese A, et al. Leukocyte CD18 monoclonal antibody worsens endotoxemia and cardiovascular injury in canines with septic shock. J Appl Physiol 1993;74:1885–1892.
49. Grover R, Zaccardelli D, Colice G, et al. An open-label dose escalation study of the nitric oxide synthase inhibitor, N(G)-methyl-L-arginine hydrochloride (546C88), in patients with septic shock. Glaxo Wellcome International Septic Shock Study Group. Crit Care Med 1999;27:913–922.
50. Hesselvik FJ, Blomback M, Brodin B, Maller R. Coagulation, fibrinolysis and kallikrein systems in sepsis: relation to outcome. Crit Care Med 1989; 17:724–733.
51. Gando S, Nanzaki S, Sasaki S, Aoi K, Kemmotsu O. Activation of the extrinsic coagulation pathway in patients with severe sepsis and septic shock. Crit Care Med 1998;26:2005–2009.
52. Fourrier F, Chopin C, Goudemand J, et al. Septic shock, multi-organ failure, and disseminated intravascular coagulation: compared to patterns of antithrombin III, protein C and protein S deficiencies. Chest 1992;101:816–823.
53. Levi M, ten Cate H, van der Poll T, van Deventer SJH. Pathogenesis of disseminated intravascular coagulation in sepsis. JAMA 1993;270:975–979.
54. Yan SB, Helterbrand JD, Hartman DL, Wright TJ, Bernard GR. Low levels of protein C are associated with poor outcome in severe sepsis. Chest 2001;120:915–922.
55. Smith OP, White B, Vaughan D, et al. Use of protein-C concentrate, heparin, and haemodiafiltration in meningococcus-induced purpura fulminans. Lancet 1997;350:1590–1593.
56. Rintala E, Seppala O-P, Kotilainen P, Pettila V, Rasi V. Protein C in the treatment of coagulopathy in meningococcal disease. Crit Care Med 1998;26: 965–968.
57. Bernard GR, Vincent JL, Laterre PF, et al. Recombinant human protein C Worldwide Evaluation in Severe Sepsis (PROWESS) study group. Efficacy and safety of recombinant human activated protein C for severe sepsis. N Engl J Med 2001;344:699–709.

58. Hampton MB, Kettle AJ, Winterbourn CC. Inside the neutrophil phagosome: oxidants, myeloperoxidase, and bacterial killing. Blood 1998;92:3007–3017.
59. Tellado JM, Christou NV. Critically ill anergic patients demonstrate polymorphonuclear neutrophil activation in the intravascular compartment with decreased cell delivery to inflammatory foci. J Leukoc Biol 1991;50:547–553.
60. Simms HH, D'Amico R. Polymorphonuclear leukocyte dysregulation during the systemic inflammatory response syndrome. Blood 1994;83:1398–1407.
61. Steinberg KP, Milberg JA, Martin TR, Maunder RJ, Cockrill BA, Hudson LD. Evolution of bronchoalveolar cell populations in the adult respiratory distress syndrome. Am J Respir Crit Care Med 1994;150:113–122.
62. Belaaouaj A, McCarthy R, et al. Mice lacking neutrophil elastase reveal impaired host defense against Gram-negative bacterial sepsis. Nat Med 1998; 4:615–618.
63. Kuang-Yao Y, Arcaroli JJ, Abraham E. Early alterations in neutrophil activation are associated with outcome in acute lung injury. Am J Resp Crit Care Med 2003;167:1567–1574.
64. Fingerle G, Pforte A, Passlick B, et al. The novel subset of CD14+/CD16+ blood monocytes is expanded in sepsis patients. Blood 1993;82:3170–3176.
65. Belge K, Dayyani F, Horelt A, et al. The proinflammatory CD14+CD16+DR++ monocytes are a major source of TNF. J Immunol 2002;168:3536–3542.
66. Geissmann F, Jung S, Littman DR. Blood monocytes consist of two principal subsets with distinct migratory properties. Immunity 2003;19:71–82.
67. Lin RY, Astiz ME, Saxon JC, et al. Altered leukocyte immunophenotypes in septic shock: studies of HLA-DR, CD11b, CD14 and IL-2R expression. Chest 1993;104:847–853.
68. Adib-Conquy M, Adrie C, Moine P, et al. NF-kB expression in mononuclear cells of septic patients resembles that observed in LPS tolerance. Am J Respir Crit Care Med 2000;162:1877–1883.
69. Stout RD, Suttles J. Functional plasticity of macrophages: reversible adaptation to changing microenvironments. J Leuk Biol 2004;76:509–513.
70. MacConmara M, Lederer JA. B cells. Crit Care Med 2005;33:S514–S516.
71. Hotchkiss RS, Tinsley KW, Swanson PE, et al. Sepsis-induced apoptosis causes progressive profound depletion of B and CD4+ T lymphocytes in humans. J Immunol 2001;166:6952–6963.
72. Meakins JL, Pietsch JB, Bubenick O, et al. Delayed hypersensitivity: indicator of acquired failure of host defenses in sepsis and trauma. Ann Surg 1997; 186:241–250.
73. Heidecke CD, Hensler T, Weighardt H, et al. Selective defects of T lymphocyte function in patients with lethal intraabdominal infection. Am J Surg 1999;178:288–292.
74. Venet F, Bohe J, Debard A-L, Bienvenu J, Lepape A, Monneret G. Both percentage of gamma-delta cells and CD3 expression are reduced during septic shock. Crit Care Med 2005;33:2836–2840.
75. Hotchkiss RS, et al. Prevention of lymphocyte cell death in sepsis improves survival in mice. Proc Natl Acad Sci U S A 1999;96:14541–14546.
76. Hotchkiss RS, et al. Adoptive transfer of apoptotic splenocytes worsens survival, whereas adoptive transfer of necrotic splenocytes improves survival in sepsis. Proc Natl Acad Sci U S A 2003;100:6724–6729.
77. Coopersmith CM, et al. Inhibition of intestinal epithelial apoptosis and survival in a murine model of pneumonia-induced sepsis. JAMA 2002;287:1716–1721.

78. Michie HR, Manogue KR, Spriggs DR, et al. Detection of circulating tumour necrosis factor after endotoxin administration. N Engl J Med 1988;318:1481–1486.
79. van der Poll T, Buller HR, ten Cate H, et al. Activation of coagulation after administration of tumor necrosis factor to normal subjects. N Engl J Med 1990;322:1622–1627.
80. Hanasaki K, Yokota Y, Ishizaki J, Itoh T, Arita H. Resistance to endotoxic shock in phospholipase A2 receptor-deficient mice. J Biol Chem 1997;272:32792–32797.
81. Beutler B, Milsark IW, Cerami AC. Passive immunization against cachectin/tumour necrosis factor protects mice from lethal effect of endotoxin. Science 1985;229:869–871.
82. Tracey KJ, Fong Y, Hesse DG, et al. Anti-cachectin/TNF monoclonal antibodies prevent septic shock during lethal bacteraemia. Nature 1987;330:662–664.
83. Opal SM, Cross AS, Kelly NM, et al. Efficacy of a monoclonal antibody directed against tumor necrosis factor in protecting neutropenic rats from lethal infection with *Pseudomonas aeruginosa*. J Infect Dis 1990;161:1148–1152.
84. Bernhagen J, Calandra T, Mitchell RA, et al. MIF is a pituitary-derived cytokine that potentiates lethal endotoxaemia. Nature 1993;365:756–759.
85. Roger T, David J, Glauser MP, Calandra T. MIF regulates innate immune responses through modulation of Toll-like receptor 4. Nature 2001;414:920–924.
86. Wang H, et al. HMG-1 as a late mediator of endotoxin lethality in mice. Science 1999;285:248–251.
87. Holmes WE, Lee J, Kuang WJ, Rice GC, Wood WI. Structure and functional expression of a human interleukin-8 receptor. Science 1991;253:1278–1280.
88. Harbarth S, Holeckova K, Froidevaux C, et al., and the Geneva Sepsis Network. Diagnostic value of procalcitonin, interleukin-6, and interleukin-8 in critically ill patients admitted with suspected sepsis. Am J Respir Crit Care Med 2001;164:396–402.
89. Chishti AD, Shenton BK, Kirby JA, Baudouin SV. Neutrophil chemotaxis and receptor expression in clinical septic shock. Intensive Care Med 2004;30:605–611.
90. Egger G, Aigner R, Glasner A, Hofer HP, Mitterhammer H, Zelzer S. Blood polymorphonuclear leukocyte migration as a predictive marker for infections in severe trauma: comparison with various inflammation parameters. Intensive Care Med 2004;30:331–334.
91. Boyd O, Grounds RM, Bennett ED. A randomized clinical trial of the effect of deliberate perioperative increase of oxygen delivery on mortality in high-risk surgical patients. JAMA 1993;270:2699–2707.
92. Rivers E, Nguyen B, Havstad S, et al. Early goal-directed therapy in the treatment of severe sepsis and septic shock. New Engl J Med 2001;345:1368–1377.
93. Hayes MA, Timmins AC, Yau EH, Palazzo M, Hinds CJ, Watson D. Elevation of systemic oxygen delivery in the treatment of critically ill patients. N Engl J Med 1994;330:1717–1722.
94. Gattinoni L, Brazzi L, Pelosi P, et al. A trial of goal-oriented hemodynamic therapy in critically ill patients. SvO2 Collaborative Group. N Engl J Med 1995;333:1025–1032.
95. Yu M, Levy MM, Smith P, Takiguchi SA, Miyasaki A, Myers SA. Effect of maximizing oxygen delivery on morbidity and mortality rates in critically ill patients: a prospective, randomized, controlled study. Crit Care Med 1993;21:830–838.
96. Shands JW Jr, McKimmey C. Plasma endotoxin: increased levels in neutropenic patients do not correlate with fever. J Infect Dis 1989;159:777–780.

97. Danner RL, Elin RJ, Hosseini JM, et al. Endotoxemia in human septic shock. Chest 1991;99:169–175.
98. Donnelly TJ, Meade P, Jagels M, et al. Cytokine, complement, and endotoxin profiles associated with the development of the adult respiratory distress syndrome after severe injury. Crit Care Med 1994;22:768–776.
99. Guidet B, Barakett V, Vassal T, et al. Endotoxaemia and bacteraemia in patients with sepsis syndrome in the intensive care unit. Chest 1994;106:1194–1201.
100. Venet C, Zeni F, Viallon A, et al. Endotoxaemia in patients with severe sepsis or septic shock. Intensive Care Med 2000;26:538–544.
101. Hurley JC. Endotoxemia and Gram-negative bacteremia as predictors of outcome in sepsis: a meta-analysis using ROC curves. J Endotoxin Res 2003;9:271–279.
102. Danner RL, Natanson C, Elin RJ, et al. *Pseudomonas aeruginosa* compared with Escherichia coli produces less endotoxemia but more cardiovascular dysfunction and mortality in a canine model of septic shock. Chest 1990;98:1480–1487.
103. Hoffman WD, Danner RL, Quezado ZM, et al. Role of endotoxemia in cardiovascular dysfunction and lethality: virulent and nonvirulent Escherichia coli challenges in a canine model of septic shock. Infect Immun 1996; 64:406–412.
104. Koike K, Moore EE, Moore FA, Read RA, Carl VS, Banerjee A. Gut ischemia/reperfusion produces lung injury independent of endotoxin. Crit Care Med 1994;22:1438–1444.
105. Charpentier C, Audibert G, Dousset B, et al. Is endotoxin and cytokine release related to a decrease in gastric intramucosal pH after hemorrhagic shock? Intensive Care Med 1997;23:1040–1048.
106. Calandra T, Glauser MP, Schellekens J, et al. Treatment of Gram-negative septic shock with human IgG antibody to Escherichia coli J5: a prospective, double-blind, randomised trial. J Infect Dis 1998;158:312–318.
107. Greenman RL, Schein RM, Martin MA, et al. A controlled clinical trial of E5 murine monoclonal IgM antibody to endotoxin in the treatment of Gram-negative sepsis: the XOMA Sepsis Study Group. JAMA 1991;266:1097–1102.
108. Schedel I, Dreikhausen U, Nentwig B, et al. Treatment of Gram-negative septic shock with an immunoglobulin preparation: a prospective, randomized clinical trial. Crit Care Med 1991;19:1104–1113.
109. Cornetta A, Baumgartner JD, Lee ML, et al. Prophylactic intravenous administration of standard immune globulin as compared with core-lipopolysaccharide immune globulin in patients at high risk of postsurgical infection. N Engl J Med 1992;327:234–240.
110. McClosky RV, Straube RC, Sanders C, et al. Treatment of septic shock with human monoclonal antibody HA-1A: a randomised, double blind, placebo controlled trial. CHESS Trial Study Group. Ann Intern Med 1994;121:1–5.
111. Angus DC, Birmingham MC, Balk RA, et al. E5 murine monoclonal anti-endotoxin antibody in gram-negative sepsis: a randomised controlled trial; E5 Study Investigators. JAMA 2000;1283:1723–1730.
112. Albertson TE, Panacek EA, MacArthur RD, et al. Multicenter evaluation of a human monoclonal antibody to Enterobacteriaceae common antigen in patients with Gram-negative sepsis. Crit Care Med 2003;31:419–427.
113. Suzuki T, Hashimoto S, Toyoda N, et al. Comprehensive gene expression profile of LPS-stimulated human monocytes by SAGE. Blood 2000;96:2584–2591.

114. Bjorkbacka H, Fitzgerald, KA, Huet F, et al. The induction of macrophage gene expression by LPS predominantly utilizes MyD88-independent signalling cascades. Physiol Genomics 2004;19:319–330.

115. Remick DG, Newcombe DE, Bolgos GL, et al. Comparison of the mortality and inflammatory response of two models of sepsis: lipopolysaccharide vs cecal ligation and puncture. Shock 2000;13:110–116.

116. Echtenacher B, Freudenberg MA, Jack RS, et al. Differences in innate defense mechanisms in endotoxaemia and polymicrobial septic peritonitis. Infect Immun 2001;69:7271–7276.

117. Haziot A, Rong GW, Lin XY, Silver J, Goyert SM. Recombinant soluble CD14 prevents mortality in mice treated with endotoxin (lipopolysaccharide). J Immunol 1995;154:6529–6532.

118. Jack RS, Fan XL, Bernheiden M, et al. Lipopolysaccharide-binding protein is required to combat a Gram-negative bacterial infection. Nature 1997;389:742–745.

119. Le Roy D, Di Padova F, Tees R, et al. Monoclonal antibodies to murine lipopolysaccharide (LPS)-binding protein (LBP) protect mice from lethal endotoxaemia by blocking either the binding of LPS to LBP or the presentation of LPS/LBP complexes to CD14. J Immunol 1999;162:7454–7460.

120. Schmicke J, Mathison J, Morgiewicz J, Ulevitch RJ. Anti-CD14 mAb treatment provides therapeutic benefit after exposure to endotoxin. Proc Natl Acad Sci U S A 1998;95:13875–13880.

121. Leturcq D, Moriarty AM, Talbott G, Winn RK, Martin TR, Ulevitch RJ. Antibodies against CD14 protect primates from endotoxin-induced shock. J Clin Invest 1996;98:1533–1538.

122. Cross A, Asher L, Seguin M, et al. The importance of a lipopolysaccharide-initiated, cytokine-mediated host defense mechanism in mice against extraintestinal invasive *Escherichia coli*. J Clin Invest 1995;96:676–686.

123. Wenneras C, Ave P, Huerre M, et al. Blockade of CD14 increases Shigella-mediated invasion and tissue destruction. J Immunol 2000;164:3214–3221.

124. Le Roy D, Di Padova F, Adachi Y, Glauser MP, Calandra T, Heumann D. Critical role of lipopolysaccharide-binding protein and CD14 in immune responses against gram-negative bacteria. J Immunol 2001;167:2759–2765.

125. Arbour NC, Lorenz E, Schutte BC, et al. TLR4 mutations are associated with endotoxin hyporesponsiveness in humans. Nat Genet 2000;25:187–191.

126. Verbon A, Dekkers PE, ten Hove T, et al. IC14, an anti-CD14 antibody, inhibits endotoxin-mediated symptoms and inflammatory responses in humans. J Immunol 2001;166:3599–3605.

127. Hagberg L, Briles DE, Eden CS. Evidence for separate genetic defects in C3H/HeJ and C3HeB/FeJ mice, that affect susceptibility to gram-negative infections. J Immunol 1995;134:4118–4122.

128. Takeuchi O, Hoshino K, Akira S. Cutting edge: TLR2-deficient and MyD88-deficient mice are highly susceptible to *Staphylococcus aureus* infection. J Immunol 2000;165:5392–5396.

129. Medvedev AE, Lentschat A, Kuhns DB, et al. Distinct mutations in IRAK-4 confer hyporesponsiveness to lipopolysaccharide and interleukin-1 in a patient with recurrent bacterial infections. J Exp Med 2003;198:521–531.

130. Hawn TR, Verbon A, Lettinga KD, et al. A common dominant TLR5 stop codon polymorphism abolishes flagellin signaling and is associated with susceptibility to legionnaires' disease. J Exp Med 2003;198:1563–1572.

131. de Groote MA, Martin MA, Densen P, et al. Plasma tumour necrosis factor levels in patients with presumed sepsis: results in those treated with antilipid A antibody vs placebo. JAMA 1989;262:249–251.
132. Calandra T, Baumgartner JD, Grau GE, et al. Prognostic values of tumour necrosis factor/cachectin, interleukin-1, interferon-alpha, and interferon-gamma in the serum of patients with septic shock. Swiss-Dutch J5 immunoglobulin study group. J Infect Dis 1990;161:982–987.
133. Marano MA, Fong Y, Moldawer LL, et al. Serum cachectin/tumour necrosis factor in critically ill patients with burns correlates with infection and mortality. Surg Gynecol Obstet 1990;170:32–38.
134. Pinsky MR, Vincent JL, Deviere J, et al. Serum cytokine levels in human septic shock: relation to multiple-system organ failure and mortality. Chest 1993;103:565–575.
135. Debets JM, Kampmeijer R, van der Linden MP, et al. Plasma tumour necrosis factor and mortality in critically-ill septic patients. Crit Care Med 1989;17:489–494.
136. Damas P, Reuter A, Gysen P, et al. Tumour necrosis factor and interleukin-1 serum levels during severe sepsis in humans. Crit Care Med 1989;17:975–978.
137. Lehmann LE, Novender U, Schroeder S, et al. Plasma levels of macrophage migration inhibitory factor are elevated in patients with severe sepsis. Intensive Care Med 2001;27:412–415.
138. Knaus WA, Harrel FE, LaBreque JF, et al. Predicted risk of mortality to evaluate the efficacy of anticytokine therapy in sepsis. Crit Care Med 1996;24:46–56.
139. Zeni F, Freeman B, Natanson C. Inflammatory therapies to treat sepsis and septic shock: a reassessment. Crit Care Med 1997;25:1095–1100.
140. van Dissel JT, van Langevelde P, Westendorp RG, Kwappenberg K, Frolich M. Anti-inflammatory cytokine profile and mortality in febrile patients. Lancet 1998;351:950–953.
141. Taniguchi T, Koido Y, Aiboshi J, Yamashita T, Suzaki S, Kurokawa A. The ratio of interleukin-6 to interleukin-10 correlates with severity in patients with chest and abdominal trauma. Am J Emerg Med 1999;17:548–551.
142. Eickacker PQ, Parent C, Kalil A, et al. Risks and the efficacy of anti-inflammatory agents:retrospective and confirmatory studies of sepsis. Am J Respir Crit Care Med 2002;166:1197–1205.
143. Girardin E, Grau GE, Dayer JM, Roux-Lombard P, Lambert PH. Tumor necrosis factor and interleukin-1 in the serum of children with severe infectious purpura. N Engl J Med 1998;319:397–400.
144. Eskandari MK, Bolgos G, Miller C, Nguyen DT, DeForge LE, Remick DG. Anti-tumor necrosis factor antibody therapy fails to prevent lethality after cecal ligation and puncture or endotoxemia.. J Immunol 1992;148:2724–2730.
145. Oberholzer A, Harter L, Feilner A, Steckholzer U, Trentz O, Ertel W. Differential effect of caspase inhibition on proinflammatory cytokine release in septic patients. Shock 2000;14:253–257.
146. Stueber F, Peterson M, Bokelmann F, et al. A genomic polymorphism within the tumour necrosis factor locus influences plasma tumour necrosis factor-alpha concentrations and outcome of patients with severe sepsis. Crit Care Med 1996;24:381–384.
147. Gordon AC, Lagan AL, Aganna E, et al. TNF and TNFR polymorphisms in severe sepsis and septic shock: a prospective multicentre study. Genes Immun 2004;5:631–640.

148. Fischer CJ Jr, Opal SM, Dhainaut JF, et al. Influence of an anti-tumor necrosis factor mononuclear antibody on cytokine levels in patients with sepsis. The CB0006 Sepsis Syndrome Study Group. Crit Care Med 1993;21:318–327.

149. Abraham E, Wunderink R, Silverman H, et al. Efficacy and safety of monoclonal antibody to human tumour necrosis factor alpha in patients with sepsis syndrome: a randomised, controlled, double-blind, multicentrer clinical trial. TNF-alpha Mab Sepsis Study Group. JAMA 1995;273:934–941.

150. Reinhart K, Wiegland-Lohnert C, Grimminger F, et al. Assessment of the safety and efficacy of the monoclonal anti-tumor necrosis factor antibody-fragment, MAK 195F, in patients with sepsis and septic shock: a multicenter, randomised, placebo-controlled, dose-ranging study. Crit Care Med 1996;24:733–742.

151. Opal SM, Fischer CJ, Dhainaut JF, et al. Confirmatory interleukin-1 receptor antagonist trial in severe sepsis. A phase III, randomized, double-blind, placebo-controlled, multicenter trial. Crit Care Med 1997;25:1115–1124.

152. Warren BL, Eid A, Singer P, et al., and the KyberSept Trial Study Group. Caring for the critically ill patient. High-dose antithrombin III in severe sepsis: a randomized controlled trial. JAMA 2001;286:1869–1878.

153. Dhainaut JF, Tenaillon A, Hemmer M, et al. Confirmatory platelet-activating factor antagonist trial in patients with severe gram-negative bacterial sepsis: a phase III, randomised, double-blind, placebo-controlled, multicentre trial. BN 52021 Sepsis Investigator Group. Crit Care Med 1998;26:1927–1931.

154. Abraham E, Reinhart K, Opal S, et al. OPTIMIST trial study group. Efficacy and safety of tifacogin (recombinant tissue factor pathway inhibitor) in severe sepsis. JAMA 2003;290:238–247.

155. Lopez A, Lorente JA, Steingrub J, et al. Multiple-centre, randomized, placebo-controlled, double-blind study of the nitric oxide synthase inhibitor 546C88: effect on survival in patients with septic shock. Crit Care Med 2004;32:21–30.

156. Ertel W, Keel M, Bonaccio M, et al. Release of anti-inflammatory mediators after mechanical trauma correlates with severity of injury and clinical outcome. J Trauma 1995;39:879–885.

157. Munford RS, Pugin J. Normal responses to injury prevent systemic inflammation and can be immunosuppressive. Am J Respir Crit Care Med 2001;163:316–321.

158. Ayala A, Song GY, Chung CS, Redmond KM, Chaudry IH. Immune depression in polymicrobial sepsis: the role of necrotic (injured) tissue and endotoxin. Crit Care Med 2000;28:2949–2955.

159. Hartemink KJ, Paul MA, Spijkstra JJ, Girbes AR, Polderman KH. Immunoparalysis as a cause for invasive aspergillosis? Intensive Care Med 2003;29:2068–2071.

160. Benjamin CF, Hogaboam CM, Kunkel SL. The chronic consequences of severe sepsis. J Leukoc Biol 2004;75:408–412.

161. Kollef MH, Sherman G, Ward S, et al. Inadequate antimicrobial treatment of infections: a risk factor for hospital mortality amoung critically ill patients. Chest 1999;115:462–474.

162. Harbarth S, Garbonio J, Pugin J, et al. Inappropriate initial antimicrobial therapy and its effect on survival in a clinical trial of immunomodulating therapy for severe sepsis. Am J Med 2003;115:529–535.

163. Leroy O, Meybeck A, d'Escrivan T, et al. Impact of adequacy of initial antimicrobial therapy on the prognosis of patients with ventilator-associated pneumonia. Intensive Care Med 2003;29:2170–2173.

164. Bochud P-Y, Bonten M, Marchetti O, et al. Antimicrobial therapy for patients with severe sepsis and septic shock: an evidence based review. Crit Care Med 2004;32:S495–S512.
165. Rello J, Ausina V, Ricart M, et al. Impact of previous antimicrobial therapy on the aetiology and outcome of ventilator-associated pneumonia. Chest 1993;104:1230–1235.
166. Kollef MH. Ventilator-associated pneumonia: a multivariate analysis. JAMA 1993;270:1965–1970.
167. Hanberger H, Garcia-Rodriguez JA, Gobernado M, et al. Antibiotic susceptibility among aerobic Gram-negative bacilli in intensive care units in 5 european countries. JAMA 1995;281:67–71.
168. Lepper PM, Held TK, Schneider EM, Bolke E, Gerlach H, Trautmann. Clinical implications of antibiotic-induced endotoxin release in septic shock. Intensive Care Med 2002;28:824–833.
169. van Saene HK, Petros AJ, Ramsay G, Baxby D. All great truths are iconoclastic: selective decontamination of the digestive tract moves from heresy to level 1 truth. Intensive Care Med 2003;29:677–690.
170. Kollef MH. Selective digestive decontamination should not be routinely employed. Chest 2003;123(5 Suppl):464S–468S.
171. de Jonge E, Schultz MJ, Spanjaard L, et al. Effects of selective decontamination of digestive tract on mortality and acquisition of resistant bacteria in intensive care: a randomised controlled trial. Lancet 2003;362:1011–1016.
172. O'Suilleabhain C, O'Sullivan ST, Kelly JL, Lederer J, Mannick JA, Rodrick ML. Interleukin-12 treatment restores normal resistance to bacterial challenge after burn injury. Surgery 1996;120:290–296.
173. Nelson S, Belknap SM, Carlson RW, et al. A randomized controlled trial of filgrastim as an adjunct to antibiotics for treatment of hospitalized patients with community-acquired pneumonia. J Infect Dis 1998;178:1075–1080.
174. Root RK, Marrie TJ, Lodato RF, et al. A multicentre, double-blind, placebo-controlled study of the use of filgrastim in patients hospitalized with pneumonia and severe sepsis. Crit Care Med 2003;31:367–373.
175. Benjamin CF, Lundy SK, Lukacs NW, Hogaboam CM, Kunkel SL. Reversal of long-term sepsis-induced immunosuppression by dendritic cells. Blood 2005;105:3588–3595.
176. Silva AT, Cohen J. Role of interferon-gamma in experimental gram-negative sepsis. J Infect Dis 1992;166:331–335.
177. Ertel W, Morrison MH, Ayala A, Dean RE, Chaudry IH. Interferon-gamma attenuates hemorrhage-induced suppression of macrophage and splenocyte functions and decreases susceptibility to sepsis. Surgery 1992;111:177–187.
178. Docke WD, Randow F, Syrbe U, et al. Monocyte deactivation in septic patients: restoration by IFN-gamma treatment. Nat Med 1997;3:678–681.
179. Houdijk AP, Rijnsburger ER, Jansen J, et al. Randomised trial of glutamine-enriched enteral nutrition on infectious morbidity in patients with multiple trauma. Lancet 1998;352:772–776.
180. Van den Berghe G, Wouters P, Weekers F, et al. Intensive insulin therapy in critically ill patients. New Engl J Med 2001;345:1359–1367.
181. Tsuneyoshi I, Yamada H, Kakihana Y, Nakamura M, Nakano Y, Boyle W 3rd. Hemodynamic and metabolic effects of low-dose vasopressin infusions in vasodilatory septic shock. Crit Care Med 2001;29:487–493.

182. Annane D, Sebille V, Charpentier C, et al. Effect of treatment with low doses of hydrocortisone and fludrocortisone on mortality in patients with septic shock. JAMA 2002;288:862–871.
183. Heyland DK, Dhaliwal R, Suchner U, Berger MM. Antioxidant nutrients: a systematic review of trace elements and vitamins in the critically ill patient. Intensive Care Med 2005;31:327–337.

4
The History of the Definition(s) of Death: From the 18th Century to the 20th Century

Leslie M. Whetstine

A person is dead when a physician says so.[1]

One of the more problematical issues in intensive care is not so much what death "is" but instead when death occurs and the operational criteria used to confirm it. This treatise will examine the history of the determination of death from the 18th century until the mid-20th century, focusing on the ways in which death has been diagnosed and misdiagnosed, the problem of premature burial, and the cultural shift that occurred when the brain death criterion was introduced.

An interesting dynamic will be shown across these time periods. Physicians in the 18th century were certain that death occurred when the heart and lungs ceased but lacked adequate tests to certify it. In the 20th century, the moment of death became less clear, and for that reason the tests physicians had finally perfected proved insufficient. This chapter lays the foundation for this dissertation and frames the question, "When is dead dead?" by discussing it in an historical sequence.

Historically, until the early 20th century, physicians' inexperience in human anatomy and physiology left them poorly equipped to accurately test for death. Despite the fact that death could not be assessed with precision instruments, the moment when an individual was considered dead was simple and absent substantial disagreement: From the 18th through mid-20th centuries, a person was declared dead when her heart stopped beating and her lungs ceased to function; this was also known as the cardiorespiratory definition of death. A consensus emerged that once the heart and lungs ceased to function the person was dead, although the empirical criteria to test for death were suspect, depending more on folklore, wives' tales, and superstition than on medical expertise. Because of this critical divide between theory and practice, instances of premature burial occurred.

Refined tests with enhanced sensitivity to measure somatic functions would come about later, in the early part of the 20th century. However, in this time period, while the criteria to test death were by now well established, the understanding of when death occurred became the subject of great debate. The fear of premature burial was replaced by the fear of suspended animation regulated

65

by life support systems. These issues culminated in the latter part of the 20th century when the cardio respiratory definition of death was reevaluated and a new notion of brain death was introduced. In addition to raising new questions as to the moment of death, the brain death criterion further necessitated that empirical tests be revised.

It is necessary to establish a working definition of death in order to explore the topics presented above. The nature of death, however, does not lend itself to one discipline; it cannot be defined without considering metaphysics, sociology, theology, and medicine. Death evades an immutable objective definition and instead is understood in subjective terms that are culturally and historically regulated.[2] Karen Gervais argues that a "decision of significance" must be established before criteria to test for the definition of death can be imposed. Such a decision identifies specific features that are necessary to differentiate a living person from a dead person and the conceptual reasons why such features are significant.[3]

Historically, the permanent cessation of heart and lung activity constituted death because the absence of heart and lung function quickly resulted in the failure of the entire organism. Thus, consensus emerged that cardiac and respiratory activities were significant for distinguishing the living from the dead. The moment of death was firmly established but the task of creating criteria to test for the permanent quiescence of these functions proved more challenging and often had devastating results.

Safeguards to prevent premature burial date back to antiquity with the Thracians, Romans, and Greeks, who each waited 3 days for putrefaction to begin before burying their dead.[4] The Romans took a more extreme approach by cutting off a finger to see if the stump bled (spilling blood would imply circulation) in addition to calling out the person's name three times while on the funeral pyre.[5] It is clear that premature burial was a concern, although it did not reach a fevered pitch until the 18th century; this was largely facilitated by the intellectual climate.

The Enlightenment and Scientific Revolution catalyzed a radical change in perceptions of life and death. Secularization, together with a mechanistic interpretation of the body and new burial practices, encouraged a sense of isolation by individualizing the person, and, subsequently, personalizing their death.[6] Belief in the afterlife was no longer as important as life in the "here and now" due in part to the works of Bacon, Descartes, and Galileo, which focused on the notion that life could be improved if not perfected by scientific manipulation. Galileo compared mastering nature with mastering mathematics. Once the patterns and rules were discovered, the argument followed that outcomes could be accurately predicted and ultimate understanding of the body could be achieved. Accordingly, there was little practical need to concern oneself with an afterlife if this life could be manipulated by the art of medicine.[7]

The revulsion against cadaveric dissection found in the 16th and 17th centuries dissipated as the study of human anatomy revealed the secrets of the "belle mécanique," or the beautiful machine.[8] Man was no longer an enigma but could be deconstructed and dutifully examined. Such knowledge revealed the unique vulnerabilities of the human body and served to heighten an awareness of oneself and one's mortality as understood within the new mechanistic paradigm. Illness could now be directly related to a particular malfunction within the individual rather than a curse or punishment for wrongdoing; sickness was no longer capricious but traced directly to one's own body.

Changes in 18th century tombstone iconography also had a profound impact on the perception on death. Effigies and plaques that accurately depicted the deceased individual now adorned individual graves.[9] Further, the introduction of the coffin meant burial was no longer a communal experience where bodies were commingled in catacombs or mausoleums, but was an isolated event, effectively sealing off the body from any other.[10] Fear of "subterranean seclusion" and premature interment became endemic due to ideological changes coupled with the uncertainty of the signs of death.[11]

The anxiety of premature burial was not simply a literary device found in the legendary works of Edgar Allan Poe, but it permeated the collective conscience as scientists began to study the phenomena of suspended animation and resuscitation. The horror of science gone awry illustrated in Mary Shelly's *Frankenstein* was based on the work of Giovanni Aldini, a physics professor in Bologna who pioneered electrical cardiac resuscitation.[12] Reality was becoming as bizarre as fiction while the line between them grew less distinct through each new medical discovery.

Knowledge of artificial respiration was well documented by the 1740s, though the first recorded incident dates back to 1627, when William Harvey maintained a decapitated rooster's lungs and circulation with a bellows.[13] Giovanni Bianchi is known for resuscitating a canine in 1755 using electricity; this technique was applied to the first human 19 years later. By the early 19th century, electroresuscitation and artificial respiration helped increase public fears of the inability to distinguish life from death and with that the hysteria of premature burial gained momentum.

It is a fact that premature burial occurred; its frequency however, is debated. Physicians had an obvious self-interest in downplaying such instances but a near universal distrust of the medical establishment bred communal hysteria. Disagreement in the medical field itself over the uncertainty of the signs of death in addition to professional insecurity further eroded the public confidence. Further challenging physicians' credibility were the abundance of charlatans and quacks, which were difficult to distinguish from physicians, especially in rural areas.[14] Despite the sensationalist headlines run by the press that "many ugly secrets are locked up underground," some physicians in the 18th and 19th centuries collected data in order to better understand the phenomenon of premature burial to prevent further occurrences as well as to bolster their status in society.[15] Jean Bruhier-d'Ablaincourt, a Paris physician, attested that 72 people were mistakenly declared dead in 1742.[16] In 1842, J. de Fontenelle reported 46 incidences of misdiagnosis of death or actual premature interment, and just 3 years later Carré recorded an additional 46 cases of persons who revived before burial.[17] In 1896, T.M. Montgomery oversaw the disinterment of the Fort Randall Cemetery. He speculated from the exhumed remains that nearly 2% of persons had been buried alive, the unfortunate victims of suspended animation.[18] M. Josat, a 19th century French physician, studied "apparent death" by chronicling how long it took for persons who were declared dead to revive. According to Josat's records, 30 persons recovered in 2 to 8 hours; 58 recovered in 8 to 15 hours; 47 recovered in 15 to 20 hours; 20 persons recovered in 20 to 36 hours; and in 7 cases 36 to 42 hours elapsed before recovery.[19] The causes of apparent death included lack of oxygen, apoplexy, hysteria, overdose, and concussion, with concussed victims reviving in the shortest amount of time.[20]

Women may have been especially vulnerable to being misdiagnosed as dead because they suffered bouts of fainting and fits of hysteria that accurately feigned death. William Tebb observed the following:

Nervous and highly hysterical females, who are subject to fainting fits are the most frequent subjects of this kind of apparent death, in which the person seems in a state very nearly resembling that of hibernating animals, such as the dormouse, bat, toad, frog, etc. which annually become insensible, motionless and apparently dead, on the setting in the winter's cold, but spontaneously revive on the returning warmth of spring. Here by some peculiar and as yet unknown circumstance, the vital principle has its action suspended, but neither its existence destroyed, nor its organs injured, so as absolutely to prevent recovery, if not too long neglected.[21]

Also, a Roman law still imposed in some areas of 18th century Europe required physicians to perform a Caesarian section on females who died in labor. If a female were hastily declared dead but in fact was not, the procedure would be deadly given the lack of antiseptics and antibiotics.[22] Advances in bacteriology would not come until the works of Pasteur and Koch in the 1860s, and sulfa drugs and antibiotics would not revolutionize the pharmacopoeia until the 20th century.[23]

There is an extensive literature on instances of premature burial ranging from ancient to contemporary times, although for the purpose at hand a brief summary of the more infamous cases will suffice. In a New York hospital in May 1864, a male patient unexpectedly died. In order to determine the cause of death a postmortem examination was ordered. When the first incision was made however, the "dead man" lunged at the physician and grasped his throat. The physician promptly died of apoplexy while the "dead man" went on to make a full recovery.[24]

Two renowned cases occurred in 17th century Scotland. Marjorie Elphinstone was declared dead and subsequently buried without incident. She revived while grave robbers attempted to steal her jewelry, and according to records, she ultimately walked home. In a similar event, Margaret Halcrow Erksime was purposely buried in a shallow grave in order for the sexton to steal her jewels. Having difficulty in obtaining a ring from her finger, the sexton began to cut the finger off, at which point the dead woman awoke and eventually recovered.[25]

Another case that is frequently cited in the literature concerns a young girl who was visiting Edisto Island, South Carolina. During her holiday she had fallen ill from diphtheria and was immediately entombed in a local family's mausoleum in order to prevent further spread of the disease. The mausoleum was reopened after the family's son was killed in the Civil War and the small skeleton was found lying next to the door.[26] The following is an excerpt from a letter published by Dr. Brouardel, the director of the Paris morgue on October 1, 1867:

I exhumed at eight p.m. Philomèle Jonetre, aged twenty-four, buried at five p.m. in a grave six feet deep. Several persons heard her tap distinctly against the lid of the coffin. These blows appeared to me to have left visible marks, but I did not hear them myself...Ammonia and other restoratives were applied...She was not dead, but like a candle, the flames of which had been extinguished, though the wick continues to glow. No definite sounds of the heart, but the eyelids moved in my presence.[27]

Perhaps the greatest risk of being buried alive occurred in times of epidemic and civil unrest. During the outbreaks of cholera, plague, and smallpox, the deceased were interred quickly for infection control. Both renowned British medical periodicals, *The Lancet* and *The British Medical Journal* (BMJ), addressed the problem of hasty interment in the late 19th century. *The Lancet* exposed a rash of premature burials resultant from the cholera outbreak. The article stressed the need to ascertain the cause and fact of death before burial and compared such "inexcusable carelessness" akin to manslaughter.[28]

The BMJ recounted a case of premature burial occurring in Naples where a female was interred while being in a state of suspended animation. The article concluded with a description of the court's penalty for the physician who signed the death certificate and the major who authorized her burial. Each was sentenced to 3 months in prison for involuntary manslaughter.[29] Many of the foremost graphic accounts of premature interment can be found in *Premature Burial and How it May be Prevented*. In it, William Tebb declares that narrow escapes from premature burial numbered in the thousands and that evidence of such occurrences could be found wherever cemeteries were removed due to overpopulation.[30] Such evidence usually involved the following: bodies flipped on their faces, the limbs broken or badly dislocated, the hair and clothing torn, and the body mutilated from the torture of entombment.[31] Tebb concluded that premature interment was vastly underreported in order to spare the family such a horrifying image of their loved one and in order for physicians to maintain public trust.[32]

Horace Welby addressed the unthinkable in his work *Mysteries of Life, Death, and Futurity* in 1861. In his chapter on trance, he concludes that suspended animation does not always lead to the suspension of consciousness; thus a person could be well aware that he or she is about to be buried alive. He supports this premise from a case where a young woman who appeared to be dead was prepared for burial. Before the coffin lid was nailed shut, however, she was observed to perspire profusely. She soon revived and retold her terrifying experience of being unable to speak or move but being able to clearly hear and feel others around her.[33]

Safeguards to prevent premature burial were creative though impractical and often bordered on the macabre. One 1790 practice in England involved laying a corpse out and painting the words "I am dead" above it in silver nitrate on a pane of glass. The silver nitrate words remained invisible until they were converted to a visible sulfide form by a surplus of hydrogen sulfide gas emitted from the corpse.[34] Once the declaration was apparent, the body was buried, though it could take some time for enough sulfide gas to accumulate.

In the early 20th century, Anthony de Chionski invented an apparatus that functioned as a vacuum chamber in which to assure death.[35] The body was placed within the chamber while air was incrementally removed; any movement of the body during the process would be cause to stop and check for signs of life. Absence of movement after undergoing the process signified that the corpse was in fact dead.

Christian Eisnebrandt invented the prototype of the "life preserving coffin" in 1843.[36] It was fashioned with wires and pins, which facilitated the lid to spring open if any movement was detected within the coffin. In 1897 Count Karnicé-Karnicki invented a similar "life signaling" coffin that would alert the outside world if the inhabitant revived.[37] The coffin was hermetically sealed and equipped with a tube approximately 3.5 inches in diameter that extended from the coffin to the surface. The tube was affixed to a spring-loaded ball, which rested upon the body's chest and would release at the slightest movement causing the lid of the box to open to allow for the passage of air and light inside. At the surface, a flag would raise while a bell would sound for 30 minutes. If the body should revive during the night, a lantern would burn as well.

A "torpedo coffin" was suggested to deter grave robbers who frequented new burial sites to pilfer corpses for jewels or other valuables. If disturbed, the torpedo coffin would emit an explosive current. Less violent means to discourage grave robbers involved sprinkling ashes over the tops of graves, which would reveal footprints.[38] A "preserver" or "corpse cooler" was favored in the later half of the 18th century, which allowed the body to putrefy while packed on ice.[39] The corpse cooler was constructed out of a wooden box with a galvanized liner. It allowed for ice to be stocked up to the body's shoulders while a glass pane allowed the face to be viewed. Openings were drilled into the cooler to facilitate a continuous ice supply while a hose aided in drainage (both for water and bodily fluid) into a bucket beneath the cooler.[40] If a corpse cooler was not on hand, the body could be placed in sod instead.[41]

The question that arises thus far is what methods were physicians using to determine death that caused such ghastly mistakes and required such extreme measures be taken? Not surprisingly, there was little agreement in the 18th and 19th centuries on which methods could accurately confirm death and the dubious process of testing could take hours. In fact, simply waiting, referred to as the Death Watch, was standard practice before accurate tests were established.[42]

Thierry pioneered the concept of waiting mortuaries, which were large rooms with glass doors where corpses were left to decay in sanitary isolation before burial.[43] The bodies were arranged in rows on sarcophagi, each one tilting downward with the deceased in a supine position.[44] An additional safeguard consisted of a ring fitted for each corpse with a string attached to it that was tied to a set of bells affixed above the head. Any movement of the body would stir the bells, which in turn alerted a caretaker, staffed 24 hours a day, to check for signs of life. Usually however, any movement was due to the build up of gasses within the body rather than revival.

The mortuary rooms were separated between the rich and poor, although aside from the types of flowers adorning the bodies, no practical difference between them existed.[45] Humane Societies to resuscitate the apparently dead were established in the 1760s and spread throughout England, the United States, the West Indies, South America, and North Africa.[46]

The London Society claimed to have resuscitated over 2000 people by 1796, although what level of functionality these individuals were returned to is not documented.[47] One of the primary problems with Humane Societies was that a person was only declared dead after failure to resuscitate. Ostensibly, this meant that there was no longer a "natural death," but death could only be declared after every medical restorative had been applied. This mentality is a precursor to the medicalization of death seen in 20th century, which will be addressed in the following chapter.

In addition to waiting mortuaries and Humane Societies, there were many notable methods used to determine death. Johannes Creve postulated that life may not be absent if the application of a sulfur and zinc arc (used to create an electrical current) caused a contraction in an exposed muscle. Dr. Josat, whom we have noted for his studies in apparent death, won first prize from the Académie de France for his invention of the nipple pincher, whose implementation certainly would rouse one from an apparent state of death.[48] In 1813, F.E. Foderé, a Paris physician, suggested drawing an incision in the left chest to manually feel if the heart was still beating.[49]

Many individuals specifically requested such tests or others like them in order to alleviate the fear of premature interment, especially because the medical community could not adopt a single authoritative test. In response to the need for a definitive test for death, the French anatomist Jean-Jaques Winslow published *The Uncertainty of the Signs of Death and the Danger of Precipitate Interments and Dissections* in 1740. Winslow favored thrusting a long needle deep under one's toenail and was also partial to burning the apparently dead through the application of a hot iron to the feet or crown of the head.[50]

Pinpricks, blood letting, or incisions were proposed but ultimately could not be relied on with absolute certainty. Winslow's student, Bruhier d'Ablaincourt, carried Winslow's ideas further and championed the Uncertainty Thesis, that is, that all signs of death were inconclusive save for putrefaction.[51]

Putrefaction was endorsed by Diderot's Encyclopédie and gained rapid acceptance by the medical and lay communities.[52] Though putrefaction did obviate the possibility of premature burial, it was not without its drawbacks. Because waiting for a body to putrefy did not require medical expertise, this further decreased confidence in physicians' abilities. Further, waiting for decomposition posed a serious health threat to the living and was not only aesthetically displeasing but also emotionally draining on families who had to bear witness to the process. Waiting for the onset of putrefaction also hindered human dissection as anatomists preferred to study the newly dead rather than decomposed bodies.[53]

The French surgeon Antoine Louis criticized the theory that putrefaction was the only certain means to determine death. His opposition was likely due to the fact that the practice fundamentally undermined the authority of physicians. Louis emphasized the need for education, especially on the "apparent" signs of death, which could include syncopy (fainting) and lethargy among others. In an effort to prove the necessity of well-trained physicians, Louis maintained that putrefaction was not an absolute sign of death because it could be confused with gangrene, which preyed on the living.[54] Louis recommended documenting changes in the eye and rigor mortis as a more accurate measure of determining death.

The infamous *Thesaurus of Horror*, authored by John Snart in 1817, catalogues other methods used to assure death including: placing a mirror to the mouth; keeping the body warm for 1 week during the Death Watch; applying acid, electricity, or warm water to the soles of the feet; placing tissue paper over the nose and mouth; pumping scotch snuff up the nose; funneling ammonia down the throat; severing the jugulars; separating the carotid arteries; cutting the medulla in half; and piercing the heart.[55] Obviously, if one was not dead before these tests were performed, one was assuredly dead afterward.

By the mid-19th century, physicians were well acquainted with thanatomeisis, or death feigning.[56] Such conditions that mimicked death included alcoholic stupor, extreme cold, opiates, hemorrhage, apoplexy (stroke), suffocation, fever, head injury, lightening strike, diabetic ketoacidosis, epilepsy, drowning, and hysterical fainting.[57] Inhalation anesthesia was introduced in 1846, which also mimicked death.

Suspended animation was problematic, and occupied much of the scientific debate over the signs of death.[58] Research on animals provided perplexing data. Scientists found that the most primitive single-celled organisms could return to life after months of apparent death and worms had the stunning ability to revive even decades after apparent death.[59] Tebb cited other instances of suspended animation in animals including pond trout and snails. The former could be frozen in snow for days but regain life when brought back to body temperature, while the latter could be dry and in a state of dormancy for 15 years but easily revived by cold water.[60]

It was not a far leap to speculate whether human beings could possess this power of "hibernation" or suspended animation similar to the states found in animals.[61] Instances of human torpor can be found in the literature concerning Indian fakirs. An Indian Sanskrit scholar was renowned for his ability for self-induced trance. Skepticism and rumors of a hoax were put to rest in 1889 when the fakir submitted to a medical exam upon entering his trance.[62]

The physician reported that the fakir's heartbeat and pulse slowly decreased until it could no longer be detected by auscultation or palpation. The fakir was wrapped in a shroud and entombed in an underground cell for a period of 33 days.[63] He was in rigor mortis when the tomb was opened and appeared on all levels to be dead. Three days later, however, the fakir was fully recovered.[64] This experiment was chilling, for it forced the question of how many other individuals could be in a similar state of life-in-death but would not be as fortunate to be exhumed.

Most 18th century physicians skilled in resuscitation believed that suspended animation was the result of a true suspension of circulation and respiration.[65] Others in the medical establishment, however, denied such a condition existed. They rejected the notion that circulation and respiration had in fact ceased and insisted that such functions were merely undetectable by standard devices.[66] The debate was settled by the late 19th century discovery of open chest cardiac massage, which could restart a heart that had ceased beating.[67]

Such discoveries allowed 19th century physicians to shed their previous image and propelled them into a secure status. Instead of developing a single test for death as Winslow attempted, physicians now relied on a variety of tests and incorporated newer ones with traditional ones.[68] In 1819, Rene Laennec had a serendipitous encounter with a portly young female patient that lead to the invention of the crude stethescope. Laennec, not wanting to place his ear to his patient's breast, rolled up his notebook and used it to amplify her heart sounds.[69] It was not until 1846, however, that Eugene Bouchut used it as a diagnostic tool to test for death.[70]

The 19th century fascination with suspended animation launched the search for more sensitive tests to determine the presence of heartbeat and circulation while traditional tests were employed as well. Tests for respiration in the 19th century included the following: a mirror held to the mouth; a feather placed under the nose; submerging the body in water for the presence of bubbles; auscultation with a stethoscope; and a hygrometer held to the nose. Tests for circulation included palpating for a pulse manually or cutting open an artery to detect the presence of flowing blood. The following empirical signs indicated circulatory failure: livid spots, pallid skin, depressed loins, sunken eyeballs, relaxed sphincter, and a cold body.[71] Carl Wunderlich was the first to measure body temperature in the 1860s and thermometers were employed from 1868 to 1880 in order to ascertain a person's "vital fire."[72]

Newer tests were more technical but also proved to be more destructive to the body. High-intensity heat lamps were used in order to view circulation through the webbing between fingers. Microphones were used in order to clearly detect chest sounds and x-ray fluoroscopy was used in order to determine movement of internal organs.[73] The ophthalmoscope was used to examine changes in the vessels of the eyes. The presence of boxcars, or stationary segments in the eye, indicated a lack of circulation and loss of cardiac activity.[74] The hypodermic syringe, having been recently improved, was used to inject ammonia into the body in order to elicit an inflammatory response. Drs. Cloquet and Laborde invented a technique where a new steel needle was inserted deep into a muscle. Their theory maintained that when inserted into living muscle the steel needle would be metabolized and rust, but when inserted into a dead muscle the needle would remain shiny and without corrosion.[75]

Other tests to check for inflammatory response were widely used. These included burning the skin over an open flame, pouring boiling water over the body, or inserting a heated cautery deep into the flesh. Dr. A.T. Middledorpf was known for inserting a needle directly into the heart with a flag attached to the other end that would ceremoniously wave if the heart were still beating.[76] The complexity of these tests elevated the status of physicians, and the fact that most of these tests would kill those who were still living did not curtail the practice.

Arterial embalming was introduced in the 1880s and 1890s and effectively squelched the fear of premature burial.[77] Embalming has been used by various cultures throughout history, but in its original form it meant to anoint with balm or natural sap.[78] Embalmment was an ancient practice that involved removing the internal organs, packing the cavities with chemical solution, and allowing the body to dehydrate, as evidenced by the ancient Egyptian mummies.

Modern arterial embalming involves replacing a body's fluids with chemicals in order to disinfect the body and slow the rate of decomposition by inhibiting the growth of microorganisms.[79] The fear of premature burial may have been the initial impetus to accept the practice because embalming is not necessary unless a body is transported over some distance.[80] Today, embalming is mainly used to prepare the body for viewing, a custom mainly practiced in the United States and Canada.

The early part of the 20th century was a somewhat awkward transition stage for medicine; however, as it enjoyed monumental successes but still retained some of its primitive roots in folklore and superstition with regard to determining death. As late as 1926, a primary text, *Medical Diagnosis for the Student and Practitioner*, shows this dichotomy:
Signs of Life in Persons Apparently Dead

1. A deep red or purple color in the fingertips will become evident gradually if a firm ligature be applied to the digit.
2. Several hours after a supposed death blood will flow persistently from a cut artery.
3. If a needle thrust into the tissues and left for a time becomes oxidized, life is present.
4. If any cloud repeatedly appears upon an ice-cold mirror held close to the mouth, there is respiration, but its absence does not alone suffice to prove death.
5. If a powerful vesicant produces redness or blisters, there is life.
6. If a body fails to take approximately the temperature of its environment forty-eight hours after apparent death there is life.
7. Pupillary response to light shows life, its absence does not prove death. Several hours after death it is affected neither by atrpin nor eserin.

8. Persistence of the red in, and visibility of the arteries of the optic disc are signs of life, as is also persistent clearness of the media, six to eight hours after death.
9. A sensitive cornea is a sign of life; absence of the corneal reflex is not a sign of death.
10. Presence of electric excitability in all muscles twenty-four hours after apparent death indicates life.[81]

Like their forefathers, 20th century physicians incorporated newfound sophisticated technology with traditional diagnostic tools. Fears of premature burial became but a historical remnant of centuries past, however, as interest in deconstructing the individual at the organ and cellular level occupied scientific inquiry. Carl Ludwig and Sydney Ringer developed perfusion techniques between 1910 and 1920.[82] Using these techniques, Alexis Carrel, the United State's first Nobel Laureate, effectively cultured cells, tissues, and organ systems outside the human body.[83] Doubtless, this epochal discovery was cause to reevaluate traditional notions of life and death. At this juncture we see a fundamental change from being unable to determine death due to medical inadequacy to being unable to determine death because of scientific advancement. By 1920 kidney transplantation had been attempted and had limited success in animals. The idea that organs could be procured from one body and function in another was previously conjured only within the realm of science fiction. Organ transplantation continued to fascinate, although it would not reach its zenith until 1968, with Christiaan Bernard, the ramifications of which will be discussed at length in the following chapter.

The principles of organ transplantation led neurologists to conclude that the brain, not the heart, was the primary seat of integrative functioning.[84] Scientists were now primed to experience a veritable renaissance within their field. Rather than pour boiling water over the patient's body to test for life, which they had done just years before, physicians now used complex devices like the electroencephalogram (EEG) to measure the brain directly.[85]

Advances in resuscitation proved to further blur the lines between life and death as the introduction of effective cardiopulmonary resuscitation (CPR) proved that death — as it had been traditionally understood — was not always irreversible.[86] Complicating conceptual matters further, by 1927 electric shock was able to reverse ventricular fibrillation and in 1940 Carrel's perfusion techniques facilitated life to be maintained in the head and body of a decapitated dog.[87]

Such progress in such a short amount of time was not without its problems. As Poe and Shelley's prose captured the climate of the 18th century, Huxley and Orwell's vision of medical progress gone awry echo contemporary concerns. Twentieth century society was now primed to embrace their newfound knowledge and equally quick to dissociate itself from the atrocities of premature burial and other follies perpetrated by medical ignorance. However, science does not exist in a vacuum; the boundaries imposed by ethics, the law, and social policy will necessarily dictate its course.

References

1. Kenneth V. Iserson, *Death to Dust* (Tuscon: Galen Press Ltd., 1994): 19.
2. Martin S. Pernick, "Back From the Grave: Recurring Controversies Over Defining and Diagnosing Death in History," *Death: Beyond Whole-Brain Criteria*, ed. Richard M. Zaner (Boston: Kluwer Academic Publishers, 1988): 17.
3. Karen Grandstrand Gervais, *Redefining Death* (New Haven: Yale University Press, 1986): 2.
4. Iserson, *Death to Dust*, 25.
5. Iserson, *Death to Dust*, 25.
6. Marc Alexander, "The Rigid Embrace of the Narrow House: Premature Burial and the Signs of Death," *Hastings Center Report* 10(1980): 27.
7. Alexander, "The Rigid Embrace," 27.
8. Alexander, "The Rigid Embrace," 27.
9. Alexander, "The Rigid Embrace," 27.
10. Alexander, "The Rigid Embrace," 27.
11. John Snart, *Thesaurus of Horror* (London, 1817): 145.
12. Pernick, "Back From the Grave," 23.
13. Stuart Youngner, Robert Arnold, and Renie Schapiro eds., *The Definition of Death Contemporary Controversies* (Baltimore: Johns Hopkins Press, 1999): 5.
14. Alexander, "The Rigid Embrace," 26.
15. Iserson, *Death to Dust*, 32.
16. Iserson, *Death to Dust*, 29.
17. Iserson, *Death to Dust*, 29.
18. Iserson, *Death to Dust*, 33.
19. Iserson, *Death to Dust*, 29.
20. Iserson, *Death to Dust*, 29.
21. William Tebb and Edward Perry Vollum, *Premature Burial and How it May be Prevented with Special Reference to Trance, Catalepsy, and other forms of Suspended Animation* (London, 1896): 121.
22. Iserson, *Death to Dust*, 29.
23. Roy Porter, *The Greatest Benefit to Mankind* (New York: W.W. Norton & Company, 1997): 10–11.
24. Iserson, *Death to Dust*, 28.
25. Iserson, *Death to Dust*, 32.
26. Margaret M. Coffin, *Death in Early America* (New York: Thomas Nelson Inc., 1976): 106.
27. Iserson, *Death to Dust*, 33.
28. "Burying Cholera Patients Alive," *The Lancet* 2(1884): 329–330.
29. "Buried Alive," *British Medical Journal* 2(1877): 819.
30. Tebb, *Premature Burial*, 64, 105.
31. Tebb, *Premature Burial*, 105.
32. Tebb, *Premature Burial*, 105.
33. Horace Welby, *Mysteries of Life, Death, and Futurity* (London, 1861): 119.
34. Iserson, *Death to Dust*, 25.
35. Iserson, *Death to Dust*, 27.
36. Coffin, *Death in Early America*, 106.
37. Iserson, *Death to Dust*, 36.
38. Coffin, *Death in Early America*, 107.

39. Coffin, *Death in Early America*, 108.
40. Coffin, *Death in Early America*, 108.
41. Coffin, *Death in Early America*, 108.
42. Michael DeVita, "The Death Watch: Certifying Death Using Cardiac Criteria," *Progress in Transplantation* 11.1(2001): 58.
43. Alexander, "The Rigid Embrace," 29.
44. Iserson, *Death to Dust*, 34.
45. Iserson, *Death to Dust*, 34.
46. Alexander, "The Rigid Embrace," 29.
47. Pernick, "Back From the Grave," 22.
48. Iserson, *Death to Dust*, 6.
49. Iserson, *Death to Dust*, 35.
50. Jean-Jacques Winslow, *The Uncertainty of the Signs of Death and the Danger of Precipitate Interment* (London, 1746): 24.
51. Alexander, "The Rigid Embrace," 26.
52. Pernick, "Back From the Grave," 21.
53. Alexander, "The Rigid Embrace," 26.
54. Alexander, "The Rigid Embrace," 26.
55. John Snart, *Thesaurus of Horror* (London: Sherwood, Neely and Jones, 1817): 145.
56. Iserson, *Death to Dust*, 26.
57. Pernick, "Back From the Grave," 23; DeVita, "The Death Watch," 58.
58. Snart, *Thesaurus of Horror*, 76.
59. Pernick, "Back From the Grave," 23.
60. Tebb, *Premature Burial*, 41, 42.
61. Tebb, *Premature Burial*, 43.
62. Tebb, *Premature Burial*, 44.
63. Tebb, *Premature Burial*, 44.
64. For further reading on the Indian fakirs, see also James Braid, *Observations on Trance, or Human Hibernation* (Churchill, 1850); *India Journal of Medical and Physical Science* 1(1836): 389.
65. Pernick, "Back From the Grave," 25.
66. Pernick, "Back From the Grave," 39.
67. Pernick, "Back From the Grave," 40.
68. Alexander, "The Rigid Embrace," 29.
69. Guenter B. Risse, *Mending Bodies, Saving Souls: A History of Hospitals* (New York: Oxford University Press, 1999): 316.
70. Pernick, "Back From the Grave," 38.
71. Pernick, "Back From the Grave," 24.
72. Pernick, "Back From the Grave," 38.
73. Pernick, "Back From the Grave," 38.
74. Iserson, *Death to Dust*, 27.
75. Pernick, "Back From the Grave," 39.
76. Pernick, "Back From the Grave," 39.
77. Iserson, *Death to Dust*, 36.
78. Iserson, *Death to Dust*, 185.
79. Iserson, *Death to Dust*, 185.
80. Iserson, *Death to Dust*, 185, 187.
81. Charles Lyman Greene, *Medical Diagnosis and the Student Practitioner* (Philadelphia: P. Blakiston's Son & Co., 1926): 1302.

82. Youngner, *The Definition of Death*, 5.
83. Pernick, "Back From the Grave," 53.
84. Pernick, "Back From the Grave," 53.
85. Pernick, "Back From the Grave," 53.
86. Pernick, "Back From the Grave," 54.
87. Pernick, "Back From the Grave," 53.

5
What It Feels Like to Live and Die on Prolonged Life Support

Justin Engleka

In recent years, medical technologies and therapies have advanced to the point where the ability to sustain life is unprecedented. In intensive care units (ICUs) around the world, advanced medical therapies are saving lives every day. Many patients who receive intensive care do recover and are able to lead fruitful, productive lives. However, a large majority of patients treated in ICUs are chronically or terminally ill and may not return to their prehospital baselines of function and quality of life.[1] A significant percentage of those patients will not even survive their hospitalization. In essence, our own medical advancements have also created a conundrum that requires more attention. Patients, families, and clinicians are facing many ethical, moral, and financial decisions with regard to therapies that prolong life. Until recently, there has not been much attention focused on the decisions that patients make in regard to proceeding with life-prolonging therapies indefinitely. There is, however, a body of literature on patients' preferences and lived experiences who survive their ICU stay.[1-4] Due to the fact that we cannot evaluate patients' experiences after they have died, we are left with applying some of those lived experiences from patients who are able to tell about them. This chapter will discuss the experiences of patients who live and die on life support.

Defining Quality of Life

The World Health Organization defines quality of life as "individuals' perception of their position in life in the context of the culture and value systems in which they live and in relation to their goals, expectations, standards and concerns."[5] Using this definition, it is easy to see why quality-of-life measures vary across different cultures and settings. However, there is an increasing awareness of these subjective issues in relation to patients who endure life-prolonging therapies. It is important to understand quality-of-life factors in relation to the use of intensive care services because these scarce resources are best suited for patients with increased chances of survival and higher levels of quality of life after treatment.[1]

Defining Life Support Measures

Patients who require prolonged life support are faced with an entirely different set of challenges than patients who are sustaining life on their own. Artificial life support measures may come in many forms: mechanical ventilation, kidney dialysis, tube feedings, and sometimes even blood transfusions. For the purpose of this review, patients who are living on prolonged mechanical ventilation will be highlighted. The reason for this selection is that prolonged mechanical ventilation is markedly different from tube feedings, blood transfusions, and even hemodialysis. Patients requiring intensive care on mechanical ventilation are much more confined and isolated than their counterparts on any of the previously mentioned therapies. One of the main problems in discussing long-term mechanical ventilation is that various authors and investigators use different definitions for long-term ventilation.[6,7] Nevertheless, we will attempt to describe some of the common themes from patients who have lived on prolonged life support and extrapolate their findings to people who have died.

Patients' Preferences Regarding Prolonged Life Support

Before we can discuss what patients endure while on prolonged life support, it is necessary to analyze the statistics on what patients favor in regard to life support measures. There are somewhat mixed reviews on what patients prefer, and variables such as age, depression, and disease state may play a vital role. Danis and colleagues[8] conducted a study of 69 patients aged <greater than> 55 years admitted to the medical or respiratory ICU for the purpose of assessing their preferences toward receiving intensive care again should the need arise. Seventy-four percent of patients were 100% willing to undergo intensive care again for as little as 1 month of time in their current health state. Only 4% of patients would refuse to go back to the ICU for any extension in life expectancy. Everhart and Pearlman[9] elicited preferences from an all-male subject base regarding preferences for resuscitation followed by mechanical ventilation given different clinical scenarios. In the current state of health scenario, 20% of patients would want mechanical ventilation for days, 23% for weeks, 7% for months, and only 10% would allow mechanical ventilation indefinitely. According to the Study to Understand Prognoses and Preferences for Outcomes and Risks of Treatment (SUPPORT), preferences for do not resuscitate (DNR) status were significantly associated with increased depressive symptoms. They found that depressed patients who had an improvement in their depression scores 2 months later had a fivefold increase in changing their preferences to wanting full cardiopulmonary resuscitation (CPR).[10] In a study of 50 patients with chronic obstructive lung disease prescribed home oxygen therapy, Stapleton and colleagues found that the majority of patients would want mechanical ventilation and CPR (63.6%). Older age was significantly associated with refusal of both treatments.[11] One of the main arguments of these findings is that we may not be able to apply these results to patients who have died on prolonged mechanical ventilation. It is quite possible that if patients knew the outcome of the interventions would be certain death, their preferences for prolonged life support may be different.

The Lived Experience in an Intensive Care Unit on Life Support

Most patients with advanced chronic illnesses or terminal illnesses suffer from at least several bothersome symptoms during their last weeks and months of life. Patients who are in ICUs and require life-sustaining support can face a plethora of additional variables. Due to invasive procedures, communication difficulties, frequent assessments, and other variables, patients in these situations are less able to convey their thoughts and concerns via normal communication. In addition, delirious patients may be completely unable to express any real insight into the frightful experiences that they encounter. Four stressors commonly identified by mechanically ventilated patients are dyspnea, anxiety, fear, and pain.[12] How patients deal with these stressors is completely variable and may depend on their mental status, cultural norms, life experiences, support networks, and communication from family and staff.

Communication Barriers

Perhaps one of the most obvious issues that arise with patients on long-term mechanical ventilation is the inability to communicate due to an endotracheal tube or tracheostomy. The ability to speak and communicate is perhaps one of the most important factors for coping and recovery in unhealthy individuals. When patients undergoing intensive care therapies are unable to communicate their needs and interact with their surroundings, they are placed at a great disadvantage. They are no longer able to express their fears, thoughts, and needs. In patients who are delirious or sedated, those feelings of normal concern can turn into fear, anxiety, and horror.

The inability to communicate comes in many forms: the inability to speak, the inability to hear, and the inability of staff to communicate effectively with the ventilated patient.[12] In fact, the inability to communicate was the second most stressful experience reported by Bergbon-Engbert and Haljamae in a study of 158 mechanically ventilated patients during treatment. The authors also reported a significant correlation with the inability to speak and other discomforts such as anxiety, fear, agony, and panic.[13]

Memory of the Intensive Care Unit Experience

Patients' perception of stressful events is highly variable and depends on a number of important factors. Even though patients may experience many different painful and stressful events, their recollection of those events is not always clear. Due to the relatively high prevalence of delirium or ICU psychosis, some or all events that occur during the last days and months in an ICU may be forgotten. The syndrome known as ICU psychosis is identified in ICU patients that present with symptoms similar to sleep deprivation, such as confusion, combativeness, hallucinations, and anxiety. The cause of ICU psychosis is a combination of factors including coping mechanisms, chronic and acute disease processes, medications, treatments, and ICU environmental factors.[12] It is worth mentioning that some patients, perhaps the sickest of ICU patients, are purposefully sedated and may not have any recall of ICU events. In one study by Rotondi and colleagues, 33% of 150 patients interviewed did not remember being in an ICU or the endotracheal tube.[14] This population of patients was interviewed after their ICU discharge. It is possible that if we applied these findings to patients that were not well enough to be discharged from the ICU and ultimately died, the incidence of amnesia could be higher.

Although the majority of patients can recall some of their ICU experience, it is possible that the most stressful experiences are likely to be most remembered. Rotondi and colleagues concluded from the study of 150 mechanically ventilated patients that subjects were more likely to remember experiences that were moderately to extremely bothersome.[14] In addition, the five experiences that bothered most patients, moderately to extremely, were trouble speaking (65%), being thirsty (62%), feeling tense (46%), not being in control (46%), and difficulty swallowing (44%).

Alterations in Sleep

When discussing the sleeping patterns of a mechanically ventilated patient, it is important to distinguish the difference between sleep and sedation. Clearly, the two are often confused, but are not the same. Sleep is a physiological state of the brain, whereas sedation can signify an artificial and augmented state of sleep. The term *sedation* can also be used to report the degree of unresponsiveness.[15] This concept is important to understand because mechanically ventilated patients are more likely to be chemically sedated.[16]

There are a number of variables that can account for the changes in sleeping patterns. In the ICU, patients must contend with frequent awakenings, medications, pain, tests, procedures, critical illness itself, and environmental factors such as noise, temperature, and light.[15] Interestingly, there are mixed results from studies that assessed the quality of sleep from mechanically ventilated patients. In one study of 239 survivors of critical illness, patients who received mechanical ventilation reported similar sleep quality with those patients who did not receive mechanical ventilation.[16] These results should be interpreted cautiously because these findings are subject to recall bias, and amnesia caused from sedatives or other causes. Alternatively, critically ill patients receiving mechanical ventilation spend a greater amount of time in stage 1 sleep, which signifies greater sleep fragmentation.[15] This finding may be a valid argument against the idea that patients requiring mechanical ventilation have sleep quality similar to patients breathing without a ventilator. In a study by Freedman and colleagues, approximately 200 patients were studied in four different ICUs. Sleep quality in the ICU was rated poorer than sleep quality at home by all subjects. In addition, patients indicated that the recording of vital signs and phlebotomy as the most disruptive environmental factors. Noise was not rated the most disruptive cause of sleep, but rather communication between staff and telemetry alarms were most problematic.[17]

Dyspnea and Ventilator Weaning

Most research on ventilator weaning includes objective data on weaning time, methods, and survival. Only a relatively small number of studies have included subjective findings from patients' own experiences. An awareness of these experiences is important for clinicians to understand so that they may apply these findings to critical care in the future.[18] Even with adequate oxygenation, patients can still feel the sensation of shortness of breath. When patients undergo weaning trials their chances of becoming dyspnic increase. In many cases, sedatives and opiates are withheld or decreased in anticipation of a weaning trial. Those same medications can often relieve the feelings of breathlessness. Therefore, patients may be at greater risk to become dyspnic when weaning trials are attempted. Many times, even patients who are deemed to be ventilator dependent will still undergo periodic ventilator weaning attempts. It is not uncommon for these patients to have many weaning trials until it truly determined that they cannot survive off of the ventilator. Finally, it is often a negotiation between the physician, patient, and family that determines the patient will no longer attempt ventilator weaning.

In a study of 10n alert patients receiving mechanical ventilation and who had failed two to five weaning attempts, mechanical ventilation was reported as a moderately fearful experience.[19] Furthermore, those patients reported loss of control felt external to themselves and an increased dependence on family and the ICU team. Finally, their feelings of hope increased with successful weaning, but feelings of hopelessness also increased when weaning attempts failed.

As previously discussed, patients tend to have greater recall of stressful ICU events. Ventilator weaning and the associated symptoms can clearly be classified as stressful events and therefore have a greater of chance of being recalled. Patients that have been able to discuss their experiences have given graphic details of their weaning experiences. In studies of patients' weaning experiences, they often complained about the readjustment in breathing pattern after being put back on the ventilator.[20] They also described unhelpful interventions from staff, such as being told to "calm down and relax." Overall, patients are left feeling frustrated and helpless.[20] Additional comments such as "breathing for my life" and "couldn't tell my brain to breathe" were given.[21] These accounts illustrate just how intense the experiences are for those requiring mechanical ventilation.

Summary

The actual lived experiences of patients who are on prolonged life support can vary significantly. It is likely that the most influential factor determining their experience is their overall level of consciousness. A significant number of patients who are "dying" on prolonged life support are comatose, semi-comatose, or purposely sedated. Therefore, these patients who are dying with an altered level of consciousness are less likely to have the same experiences as patients with a full range of cognition. Ultimately, we are forced to extrapolate these lived experiences to patients who actually die on life support measures.

It is quite clear that patients who require prolonged life support are among the sickest of patients in most hospitals. Furthermore, these same patients utilize a disproportionate amount of healthcare resources. Although critical care and life support measures are clearly indicated for most ICU patients, there is still a select population of patients that are unmistakably "dying" on prolonged life support. For these patients, it is somewhat unclear how they arrive at that place in time. Perhaps it is a combination of their own wishes to live a prolonged life, with the support of their families and physicians. Regardless, healthcare practitioners are often faced with many moral and ethical dilemmas on how to best care for patients that have little to no chance of survival. There are countless anecdotal experiences of patients and families who are hoping for a miracle or do not want to give up hope. These pleas for continued care are emotional and difficult to deal with in real-life situations. Finally, we are in great need of further qualitative research that examines the real-life experiences of patients who are dying on prolonged life support.

References

1. Mendelsohn AB, Chelluri L. Interviews with intensive care unit survivors: assessing post-intensive care quality of life and patients' preferences regarding intensive care and mechanical ventilation. Crit Care Med 2003;31:400–406.
2. Mendelsohn AB, Belle SH, et al. How patients feel about prolonged mechanical ventilation 1 year later. Crit Care Med 2002;30:1439–1445.
3. Fakhry SM, Kercher KW, Rutledge R. Survival, quality of life, and charges in critically ill surgical patients requiring prolonged ICU stays. J Trauma 1996;41:999–1007.
4. Douglas SL, Daly BJ, Gordon N, Brennan PF. Survival and quality of life: short-term versus long-term ventilator patients. Crit Care Med 2002;30:2655–2662.
5. WHOQOL Group: The World Health Organization Quality of Life Assessment (WHOQOL): position paper from the World Health Organization. Soc Sci Med 1995;41:1403–1409.

6. Nasraway SA, Button GJ, Rand WM, Hudson-Jinks T, Gustafson M. Survivors of catastrophic illness: outcome after direct transfer from intensive care to extended care facilities. Crit Care Med 2000;28:19–25.

7. Chatila W, Kreimer DT, Criner GJ. Quality of life in survivors of prolonged ventilatory support. Crit Care Med 2001;29:737–742.

8. Danis M, Patrick DL, Southerland LI, et al. Patients' and families' preferences for medical intensive care. JAMA 1988;260:797–802.

9. Everhart MA, Perlman RA. Stability of patient preferences regarding life-sustaining treatments. Chest 1990,97:159–164.

10. Rosenfeld KE, Wenger NS, Phillips RS, et al. Factors associated with change in resuscitation preference of seriously ill hospitalized patients: the SUPPORT Investigators; Study to Understand Prognoses and Preferences for Outcomes and Risks of Treatment. Arch Intern Med 1996;156:1558–1564.

11. Stapleton RD, Nielsen EL, Engleberg RA, Patrick DL, Curtis R. Association of depression and life-sustaining treatment preferences in patients with COPD. Chest 2005;127:328–334.

12. Thomas LA. Clinical management of stressors perceived by patients on mechanical ventilation. Adv Pract Acute Crit Care 2003;14:73–81.

13. Bergbom-Engberg I, Haljamae H. Assessment of patients' experience of discomforts during respirator therapy. Crit Care Med 1989;17:1068–1072.

14. Rotondi AJ, Chelluri L, et al. Patients' recollections of stressful experiences while receiving prolonged mechanical ventilation in an intensive care unit. Crit Care Med 2002;30:746–752.

15. Parthasarathy S. Sleep during mechanical ventilation. Curr Opin Pulm Med 2004;10:489–494.

16. Cooper AB, Thornley KS, Young GB, et al. Sleep in critically ill patients requiring mechanical ventilation. Chest 2000;117:809–818.

17. Freedman NS, Kotzer N, Schwab RJ. Patient perception of sleep quality and etiology of sleep disruption in the intensive care unit. Am J Respir Crit Care Med 1999;159:1155–1162.

18. Cook DJ, Meade MO, Perry AG. Qualitative studies on the patient's experience of weaning from mechanical ventilation. Chest 2001;120:469S–473S.

19. Lowry LW, Anderson B. Neuman's framework and ventilator dependency: a pilot study. Nurs Sci Q 1993;6:195–200.

20. Jablonski RS. The experience of being mechanically ventilated. Qual Health Res 1994;4:186–207.

21. Jenny J, Logan J. Caring and comfort metaphors used by patients in critical care. J Nurs Scholarsh 1996;28:349–352.

6
Who's in Charge in the Intensive Care Unit?

Anthony L. DeWitt

> The logical corollary of the doctrine of informed consent is that the patient generally possesses the right not to consent, that is, to refuse treatment.[1]

Every competent patient has the right to decide what will and what will not be done to him or her.[2] As one jurist put it, "Every human being of adult years and sound mind has a right to determine what shall be done with his own body, and a surgeon who performs an operation without his patient's consent commits an assault, for which he is liable in damages."[3] When a patient is alert, of sound mind, competent, and able to make his or her own decisions, there is no question that the physician must follow that person's directions even if the ultimate outcome — death — is not the result that the physician or health care organization desires or intends.[4]

Few areas, however, get so sticky as the end-of-life decision making in cases where the patient, either because of their disease process, or because of the suddenness with which their condition has been brought on (e.g., car accident, stroke, etc.), has (1) failed to make his wishes known and (2) failed to appoint anyone officially to act on his behalf.[5] When these situations present, the only safe approach for the physician and healthcare entity is to undertake judicial intervention so as to prevent claims that they failed to protect their patient from harm.[6]

Consider D.T., a gentleman who is currently the subject of litigation in Missouri. D.T. was checked into a nursing home by his second wife against the wishes of his three adult children, who wanted to bring him to a nursing home closer to their home. D.T., though competent, didn't want to ignite a family battle, and acceded to the wishes of his wife. Over the course of several months D.T. received shockingly poor care in the nursing home, and was treated as a hospice patient even though he had undergone placement of an automatic defibrillator only a few months before he was admitted to the nursing home. His weight dropped 30 pounds over 2 months, and the children frequently found him incoherent from Marinol intoxication. When he was finally transferred from the nursing home to the local hospital, the hospital physician was presented with a dilemma. The wife, who had placed him in the nursing home and who held the durable power of attorney, was under the influence of narcotics and could not lawfully consent to the procedures that needed to be performed. Instead of seeking a judicial order to determine the proper course of action, the doctor relied on the wife's daughter (who was not the child of D.T.) and permitted the patient to expire.

Under Missouri law, the children are members of the class who may bring an action for wrongful death,[7] and so the children sued for wrongful death, at least in part because they were contacted or involved in the decisionmaking process, and because the durable power of attorney was simply invalid under the situation.

If all family members are in agreement as to the proper course of action, and the physician is certain that all members are present and are voicing their concerns, then it may be appropriate to act on those requests provided someone provides the information and obtains the consent of the family members present, preferably in writing. But where family members are not in agreement, where there is disagreement about futility or continued treatment or religious beliefs or any of the other myriad concerns that attend death, the physician and healthcare entity must be very careful about acting without some legal authority.[8]

Under the law, there is a hierarchy with regard to decision making, and a process by which decisions in that process can be reviewed and forestalled. This was demonstrated repeatedly in the matter of Terry Schiavo.[9] Schiavo can really be seen as much as a failure of the legal and political systems as it can a relevant case on end of life.[10] In the latter days of her existence,[11] Schiavo became a political football as legislators, congressmen, governors, senators, and finally the Supreme Court opted to interfere or step aside as each felt appropriate.[12] The object for the healthcare provider is to steer clear of such a Shiavo-like debacle.

The hierarchy can be demonstrated by Figure 6-1.

The law prefers the competently expressed wishes of the competent patient, acting on his own, to state what his wishes are, and what he wants done [*Cruzan V. Director, MDH*, 497 U.S. 261 (1990)]. States, however, often place obstacles in the way of the patient. In the celebrated Nancy Beth Cruzan case, the Missouri Supreme Court decided that a competent person's wishes about the end-of-life care they receive must be proved by clear and convincing evidence before life support can be withdrawn.

In casting the balance between the patient's common law right to refuse treatment/ constitutional right to privacy and the state's interest in life, we acknowledge that the great majority of courts allow the termination of life-sustaining treatment. …

The common law **right** to refuse treatment is not absolute. It too must be balanced against the state's interest in **life** ….

We find no principled legal basis that permits the coguardians in this case to choose the death of their ward. In the absence of such a legal basis for that decision and in the face of this State's strongly stated policy in favor of life, we choose to err on the side of life, respecting the rights of incompetent persons who may wish to live despite a severely diminished quality of life. [*Cruzan v. Harmon*, 760 S.W.2d 408, *affirmed on appeal*, 497 U.S. 261 (1990)]

Because there was such confusion, and indeed, so many difficult decisions being foisted off on surrogate decision makers after sudden trauma, legislative

Permitted   Preferred Decisionmaker

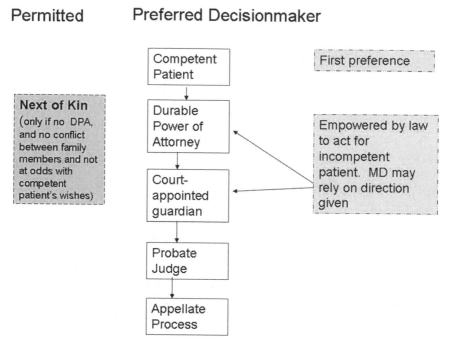

FIG. 6-1. The hierarchy of decision makers at the end of life

bodies began to adopt an old tool, the "power of attorney," to the end-of-life decisionmaking process. By creating a Durable Power of Attorney for Health Care (DPAHC), every person can specify whom he or she wants to make their end-of-life decisions on their behalf by appointing an "agent" for that purpose.[13] That agent is empowered under state law to act as fully as if the competent person herself were making the decisions. Under Missouri law, for example, a holder of a durable power of attorney is authorized to hire and fire medical personnel — a right thought necessary when religious-based facilities refused to carry out termination of life support decisions on behalf of family members. The holder of the power may require that a patient be transferred to another facility or have another physician act to end life support. Ideally, a DPAHC is coupled with a statement of wishes that are nonbinding on the DPAHC. In other words, while the principal may state their preference is not to receive a feeding tube, the DPAHC may override that decision if, in the agent's view, that is what the patient would have wanted. But where the patient is still competent, the agent has only the power that the principal (patient) gives her, and she cannot superintend a competent patient's decisions.[14]

Occasionally the situation presents where a patient is not certified as incompetent, but the agent under the DPAHC attempts to act for the patient anyway. This is another area where the law has not dealt with the conflict. Unless there is a medical certification in the file that the patient is not competent, the hospital should not act on the wishes of the agent where they contradict the wishes of the patient.

Rarely there will be situations where agents are appointed, but their decisions, when viewed by other family members, are inconsistent with what the patient is thought to want. In those situations the family members can reach around the durable power of attorney by requesting the appointment of a guardian and conservator.[15] In most states all that must be done is for one family member or "interested party" (e.g., nursing home administrator) to file a petition for appointment of guardian. The petition for guardianship is served on the patient (even where the patient may be comatose) and a guardian ad litem is appointed by the court to act on the ward's behalf. The guardian advocates for the best interest of the ward, and if the patient is competent, and willing to act on their own, generally the guardian ad litem must advocate against the guardianship. If the ward is incompetent, and this can be established by medical testimony, then the guardian ad litem must advocate for the best interests and assist the court in choosing the best guardian from the family members or interested persons. In some cases, where there are warring factions among family members, the Public Administrator is appointed to prevent one party or the other from acting against the best interests of the ward.[16]

As the Schiavo case aptly demonstrated, however, mere appointment of the guardian does not establish that there will never be challenges to the guardian's authority to authorize health care decisions. In *Schiavo*, several appeals were taken to the state appellate courts in Florida. In the end, even the appellate judges were tired of hearing the case:

Robert and Mary Schindler, the parents of Theresa Marie Schiavo, appeal the trial court's order denying their motion for relief from judgment filed pursuant to Florida Rule of Civil Procedure 1.540(b)(4). This case has an extensive legal history,17 and this is not the first motion that the Schindlers have filed seeking relief from the trial court's judgment.

The trial court entered the judgment in February 2000 following an extensive trial. The trial court determined, based on clear and convincing evidence, that Theresa Schiavo was in a persistent vegetative state and that she herself would elect to forego further use of a feeding tube. This court affirmed that judgment. *See In re Guardianship of Schiavo*, 780 So.2d 176 (Fla. 2d DCA 2001) (*Schiavo I*).

As a result of an earlier motion for relief from judgment, we required the trial court to reconfirm that medical science offered no meaningful treatment for her condition. *In re Guardianship of Schiavo*, 800 So.2d 640 (Fla. 2d DCA 2001) (*Schiavo III*). The trial court decided not only to reconfirm that issue but also to review its earlier decision that Mrs. Schiavo was in a persistent vegetative state. Following another extensive hearing at which many highly qualified physicians testified, the trial court denied the motion for relief from judgment. This court affirmed that decision. *In re Guardianship of Schiavo*, 851 So.2d 182 (Fla. 2d DCA 2003) (*Schiavo IV*).

The trial court's decision does not give Mrs. Schiavo's legal guardian the option of leaving the life-prolonging procedures in place. No matter who her guardian is, the guardian is required to obey the court order because the court, and not the guardian, has determined the decision that Mrs. Schiavo herself would make. [*Schindler v. Schiavo*, 2005 WL 600377 (Fla. App. 2 Dist.).]

Most cases do not become debacles of the Schiavo variety in large measure because physicians do such a good job of frankly explaining end-of-life options and realistic chances of recovery. However, beyond the simple question of "Who's in charge?" that the *Cruzan* and *Schiavo*-type cases establish, there risks a less understood peril.

Frequently physicians and healthcare workers provide information and help families make decisions by relying solely on the next of kin. This may be the son, the daughter, the wife, the husband, or parent of the trauma or disease victim. In 99% of the cases, these are the proper parties because these persons have the best interests of the patient at issue. But simply because a person may be the next of kin does not mean that attending to their wishes in some ways exempts a physician from a claim of medical negligence for acting on those wishes.

Under most state statutes governing wrongful death, there are a wider number of persons who can maintain an action for wrongful death than simply the most vocal next of kin. For example, under Missouri law, where a female wage earner with two children dies, leaving a husband, children, and living parents, any of those individuals can maintain an action for wrongful death. This creates a potential trap for the unwary.

Where there is any concern, expressed by the family or not, that there may be medical error in the care of a patient who is facing end-of-life decisions, it is a good idea to gather as many relatives as possible and make sure that everyone is on the same page with respect to end-of-life decision making.

A frequent concern among family members who cannot make it to the hospital in time to be included in such determinations is that they were provided with less information than they needed to make an informed decision, or more often, that medical providers were not frank in discussing causes and outcomes.

A quick return to the case of D.T. shows why it is important to include as many family members as possible. Had the natural children of D.T. (and not the stepdaughter of D.T.) been asked whether to continue life support, and try to reverse the process of organ failure, they would likely have advocated strongly to employ heroic measures. When they are not given the opportunity, it begins to look a great deal like a conspiracy between the caregivers. This resulted in charges of civil conspiracy, wrongful death, and violations of patient's rights litigation being filed against several of the healthcare providers in that case. While the case remains in litigation, and the outcome far from certain at this point, the moral of the story is clear. The greater the number of family members, the greater the number of persons who should be consulted in reaching end-of-life decisions.

References

1. *Cruzan v. Director,* Missouri Department of Health, 497 US 261 (1990).
2. *End-Of-Life Care: Forensic Medicine V. Palliative Medicine,* 31 J.L. Med. & Ethics 365 (2003 WL 23114200).

3. *Schloendorff v. Society of New York Hospital*, 211 N.Y. 125, 129-30, 105 N.E. 92, 93 (1914).
4. Brief of Amici Curiae not dead yet et al., Jeb Bush v. Michael Schiavo, 20 Issues L. & Med. 171 (2004 WL 3135533). See also *A Line Already Drawn: The Case For Voluntary Euthanasia After The Withdrawal Of Life-Sustaining Hydration And Nutrition*, 38 Colum. J.L. & Soc. Probs. 201 (2004 WL 3113773).
5. *Durable Powers Of Attorney—They Are Not Forms!* 24 Tax Mgmt. Est. Gifts & Tr. J. 211 (1999).
6. Limiting A Surrogate's Authority To Terminate Life-Support For An Incompetent Adult, 79 N.C. L. Rev. 1815 (2001 WL 1628930).
7. § 537.080 R.S.Mo. (2004) states "Whenever the death of a person results from any act, conduct, occurrence, transaction, or circumstance which, if death had not ensued, would have entitled such person to recover damages in respect thereof, the person or party who, or the corporation which, would have been liable if death had not ensued shall be liable in an action for damages, notwithstanding the death of the person injured, which damages may be sued for: (1) By the spouse or children or the surviving lineal descendants of any deceased children, natural or adopted, legitimate or illegitimate, or by the father or mother of the deceased, natural or adoptive; (2) If there be no persons in class (1) entitled to bring the action, then by the brother or sister of the deceased, or their descendants, who can establish his or her right to those damages set out in section 537.090 because of the death."
8. *Death and Dying: Opposing Viewpoints*, (Reviewed), 19 Issues L. & Med. 310 (2004 WL 1241810).
9. *In re Guardianship of Schiavo*, 792 So.2d 551 (Fla. App. 2. Dist., 2001).
10. Manuel Roig-Franzia, *Long Legal Battle Over as Schiavo Dies*, Washington Post, Apr. 1, 2005, found at http://www.washingtonpost.com/wp-dyn/articles/A15423-2005Mar31.html. See also Dynamic Complementarity: Terri's Law And Separation Of Powers Principles In The End-Of-Life Context, 57 Fla. L. Rev. 53 (2005 WL 15314).
11. Autopsy results have indicated that Terry Shiavo was not capable of thought at the end of her existence, and thus, this author does not believe that she had "life" as that term is commonly used. She was biologically interacting with her environment; nothing more.
12. Roig-Franzia, *supra*, note 10.
13. Advance Directives: Taking Control Of End-Of-Life Decisions, 14 St. Thomas L. Rev. 5 (2001 WL 1556169); Advance Medical Directives And The Authority To Compel Medical Treatment, 29 Colo. Law. 59 (Mar 2000).
14. Assessing Competence to Consent to Treatment: A Guide for Physicians and Other Health Professionals, (Reviewed), 28 J. Psychiatry & L. 281 (2000).
15. A guardian is charged with looking out for the patient's needs and welfare, and is empowered to make medical decisions. A conservator is limited to looking after and "conserving" the patient's funds and property. A conservator is not empowered to make healthcare decisions unless the order granting the conversatorship specifically states.
16. Had a Public Administrator been appointed in the Schiavo case early on, it would have ended without fanfare many years earlier.
17. See *In re Guardianship of Schiavo*, No. 90-2908-GD, 1996 WL 33496839 (Fla. Pinellas Cir. Ct. Feb. 11, 2000) (order authorizing discontinuation of artificial life support); *In re Guardianship of Schiavo*, 780 So.2d 176 (Fla. 2d DCA 2001)

(*Schiavo I*), *review denied*, 789 So.2d 348 (Fla. 2001); *In re Guardianship of Schiavo*, 792 So.2d 551 (Fla. 2d DCA 2001) (*Schiavo II*); *In re Guardianship of Schiavo*, 800 So.2d 640 (Fla. 2d DCA 2001) (*Schiavo III*), *review denied*, 816 So.2d 127 (Fla. 2002); *Schindler v. Schiavo ex rel. Schiavo*, 829 So.2d 220 (Fla. 2d DCA 2002) (table citation denying motion); *In re Guardianship of Schiavo*, No. 90-2908-GD-003, 2002 WL 31876088 (Fla. Cir. Ct. Nov. 22, 2002); *In re Guardianship of Schiavo*, No. 90-2908-GB-003, 2002 WL 31817960 (Fla. Cir. Ct. Nov. 22, 2002); *Schiavo v. Schiavo*, No. 8:03-cv-1860-T-26TGW, 2003 WL 22469905 (M.D.Fla. Sept. 23, 2003); *In re Guardianship of Schiavo*, 851 So.2d 182 (Fla. 2d DCA 2003) (*Schiavo IV*), *review denied*, 855 So.2d 621 (Fla. 2003); *Schindler v. Schiavo*, 865 So.2d 500 (Fla. 2d DCA 2003) (table decision denying prohibition); *Advocacy Ctr. for Persons with Disabilities, Inc. v. Schiavo*, 17 Fla. L. Weekly Fed. D291, 2003 WL 23305833 (M.D. Fla. Oct. 21, 2003); *Schiavo v. Bush*, No. 03-008212-CI-20, 2003 WL 22762709 (Fla.Cir.Ct. Nov. 4, 2003); *Bush v. Schiavo*, 861 So.2d 506 (Fla. 2d DCA 2003); *Schiavo v. Bush*, No. 03-008212-CI-20, 2004 WL 628663 (Fla. Cir. Ct. 2004); *Bush v. Schiavo*, 866 So.2d 136 (Fla. 2d DCA 2004); *Schindler v. Schiavo*, 866 So.2d 140 (Fla. 2d DCA 2004); *Bush v. Schiavo*, 871 So.2d 1012 (Fla. 2d DCA 2004); *Schiavo v. Bush*, No. 03-008212-CI-20, 2004 WL 980028 (Fla.Cir.Ct. May 5, 2004); *Bush v. Schiavo*, 885 So.2d 321 (Fla. 2004), *cert. denied*, — U.S. —, 125 S.Ct. 1086, — L.Ed.2d — (2005); *Schindler v. Schiavo*, No. 2D04-3451, — So.2d —, 2004 WL 2726107 (Fla. 2d DCA Nov. 24, 2004) (table decision); *In re Guardianship of Schiavo*, No. 90-2908-GD-003, 2005 WL 459634 (Fla. Cir. Ct. Feb. 25, 2005).

7
Dealing with Difficult Surrogates

Erring on the Side of Autonomy

David W. Crippen

It is difficult to count the number of times house staff have paged me frantically to say that a moribund patient's family continues to desire "everything done" despite pleas for comfort measures. This situation usually occurs at three in the morning and frequently involves an elderly patient who has been transferred from a skilled nursing facility to the hospital for recurring decompensations. There is rarely evidence in the chart of any discussion regarding end-of-life care. A phone call to the relatives of the patient invariably yields the reply, "We want everything done."

My usual response to the paging resident is that physicians are not required to do everything possible in the face of an inevitable death spiral. We are not required by any canon of ethics to render care that will not be beneficial to the patient or will not reverse the progression toward death. We are, however, required to do everything reasonable, including instituting palliative measures to avoid pain and suffering. This revelation is usually greeted with a plaintive wail, "But they want everything done!" So 45 minutes of useless cardiopulmonary resuscitation is commenced, until it is obvious that nothing more can be done.

In the United States, healthcare consumers are granted broad powers of choice with regard to health care.[1] When consumers choose to equate maintenance of vital signs (blood pressure, heartbeat, and respiration) with sapient life, physicians are not normally empowered to question this decision.[2] Critical care personnel can maintain vital signs almost indefinitely, and the public knows this. However, the odds of meaningful recovery in such cases are exceedingly small — sometimes less than the odds of winning a lottery jackpot. The media, which relentlessly broadcast emotion-laden stories of recovery and which fail to acknowledge that these stories are newsworthy precisely because they are so rare, ignores this harsh reality.

The media love the unexpected survivor, especially when long lines of experts have prophesied the person's demise.[3] As a result of all this media attention to remote possibilities, the urban legend of the "long-shot survivor" figures into our definitions of futility.[4] It might fairly be asked, "So what is wrong with lottery jackpot odds if the alternative is certain death?" The answer is that the cost of the ticket in such cases — days, weeks, or even years of futile care — is a bankrupting one, both financially and ethically. What is more, those bank-rupted are not just the patients or families who demand such care, but also the community and the medical staff who are forced to deliver it. Even the wildest optimist can see the difference between spending a dollar on a chance at millions and spending half a subsistence income on a long shot.

Most end-of-life problems facing clinicians revolve around the practical definition of futility. In the intensive care unit (ICU), life support is effective in maintaining life if life is defined as the presence of stable vital signs. Some treatments such as dialysis and mechanical ventilation may support open-ended goals of hope while at the same time prolonging open-ended suffering. Such uses of treatments are a perversion of the modalities, which were developed as a bridge between organ failure and restoration of health — or, at a minimum, extension of life, albeit life of a much lower quality. These treatments were not developed to indefinitely extend the moribund state of the actively dying. As things stand now, virtually any treatment is fair game as long as "life" is supported. If surrogates feel that a treatment can prolong vital signs during the search for a miracle — for a long-shot cure — physicians feel obliged to provide it, because under the strictest definition the treatment is not futile.[5]

Most surrogates listen to reason, but they do not have to. Most rational surrogates are unwilling to continue life support after a reasonable trial has resulted in diminishing returns, but they do not have to. The current case law is on their side. The courts have affirmed the authority of competent patients (and their surrogates by proxy) to regulate their medical treatment, regardless of their reasoning,[6] without any consideration being given to the burden of the costs to others.

Other than the expectation of a long-shot cure, there are several reasons patients and especially their surrogates demand open-ended treatment that only prolongs suffering:

1. Surrogates do not recognize suffering as such. Moribund ICU patients are usually either sedated or unresponsive. Once life-supporting care is insti-tuted, even actively dying patients look comfortable. They are pink and warm, and a constant stream of vital sign data on a monitor affirms some kind of acceptable existence. Surrogates are lulled into a perception that would not ensue were the same patient viewed in a morgue, even though the person might be equally dead or nearly so.[7] As long as the patient gives the appearance of viability and comfort, it is much more emotionally chal-lenging to accept the clinical reality of death. If the patient can just be maintained comfortably long enough, a cure is possible, if not inevitable. If the patient is dead, nothing more is possible. One of the few unarguable advantages of death in such situations is its absolute finality.

2. Physician services are no longer a controlled monopoly. There is an over-supply of physicians and there is competition for paying customers. Therefore, surrogates are in the position of being buyers in a consumers' market. Health services consumers are encouraged by the media to shop wisely, as if they were looking for a home remodeling contractor. They can and do take their

business elsewhere if they are not satisfied. Physicians thus do not necessarily serve as authorities but rather offer choices geared to customer satisfaction. By asking surrogates to make a choice in such situations, we imply that their authority in making choices extends to making bad choices.

3. As a general rule, physicians do not have an exceptional track record in explaining end-of-life issues to patients and their families.[8] The language they use and the subliminal signals they send to patients and surrogates sometimes engender ambivalence and false hope that create a demand for futile treatments. In other instances, critical care physicians may telegraph that they want death to come soon so that the bed can be available for another patient. They may rush families into doing their bidding. It is not uncommon for physicians to ask loaded questions in their quest for end-of-life decisions: "This is your grandmother's 17th transfer from a skilled nursing facility in 3 months for sepsis and respiratory failure. Now she's in kidney failure as well. What do you want to do: do everything or let her die?" Given that choice, most surrogates opt for doing something rather than nothing, even if that something perpetuates open-ended pain and discomfort.

4. The popular media, especially the tabloids, frequently feature anecdotal articles about patients who have awakened after years of coma.[9] Most, if not all, of these patients' conditions have been embellished to generate public interest, and frequently, subsequent investigators cannot find these patients. This kind of reckless journalism may be viewed simply as entertainment devoid of factual content. However, it is important to realize that the *National Enquirer*[10] is the most read newspaper in the United States and that many, if not most, of those who read it cannot distinguish between the fact and fiction printed side by side. There is nothing so strong as external validation of a deeply cherished belief. In such cases of intense desire fueled by fear and grief, even rational minds can be deceived by an unsubstantiated (or even patently false) interpretation of hope. Accordingly, some families feel that if life support systems can maintain vital signs for a day or a week, suspended animation should be possible indefinitely and should be continued until a cure is found — just as it is in tabloid tales where persistence against the odds and against all medical wisdom pays off.

5. Hospital ethics committees and palliation services are highly weighted in favor of competence to make medical decisions rather than the rationality or morality of such decisions. These entities normally go to great lengths to determine whether decision makers fit the traditional definitions of authoritative and authentic surrogates. Once authenticity and authority are determined, these services and committees usually rubber-stamp surrogates' decisions, reaffirming that no one should interfere with family dynamics. When it comes to end-of-life issues, ethics committees do not ask for consensus — they ask for consent. This attitude reaffirms surrogates' determination to tread the path of least emotional trauma and continue the search for a long-shot cure.

Because of the lack of accountability and rationality in decision making, the only indication for admitting a patient to an ICU is the media-fueled belief that application of the most sophisticated technology that critical care medicine has to offer will translate into a chance for a cure. In such a system, there are many, many more reasons to maintain warm cadavers than to make difficult decisions that result in transport to the morgue. But the fact is, slowing an inevitable death spiral means patient suffering — an unintended consequence of end-of-life care.[11]

Irrational striving for the improbable can leave the patient in perpetual suffering, without the outlet of death, a mercy that has been denied him or her. There are far worse things than death, and many of these things occur in ICUs when futility maxims are circumvented to preserve patient autonomy. There is a population of ICU patients who will die, or remain painfully moribund or vegetative, no matter what treatment is rendered. Medically inappropriate care causes pain, suffering, and discomfort — not only for the patient, but also ultimately for the family, the medical staff caring for the patient, and society at large. The fundamental maxim for these patients should be "care as comfort." Extraordinary life support for patients who will nevertheless die does not equal comfort care and should never be confused with it.

References

1. Lynn J, Teno JM, Phillips RS, et al. Perceptions by family members of the dying experience of older and seriously ill patients. SUPPORT Investigators. Study to Understand Prognoses and Preferences for Outcomes and Risks of Treatments. Ann Intern Med 1997;126:97–106.
2. Doig C, Murray H, Bellomo R, et al. Ethics roundtable debate: patients and surrogates want 'everything done' — what does 'everything' mean? Crit Care 2006;10:231.
3. Shepherd L. Shattering the neutral surrogate myth in end-of-life decision making: Terri Schiavo and her family. Spec Law Dig Health Care Law 2006;327:9–29.
4. Buckley T, Crippen D, DeWitt AL, et al. Ethics roundtable debate: withdrawal of tube feeding in a patient with persistent vegetative state where the patients wishes are unclear and there is family dissension. Crit Care 2004;8:79–84.
5. Crippen D, Hawryluck L. Pro/con clinical debate: life support should have a special status among therapies, and patients or their families should have a right to insist on this treatment even if it will not improve outcome. Crit Care 2004;8:231–233; discussion, 231–233.
6. Cranford RE. Helga Wanglie's ventilator. Hastings Cent Rep 1991;21:23–24.
7. Whetstine LM. An examination of the bio-philosophical literature on the definition and criteria of death; when is dead 'dead' and why some donation after cardiac death donors are not [dissertation]. Pittsburgh: Duquesne University; 2006.
8. Levy MM, McBride DL. End-of-life care in the intensive care unit: state of the art in 2006 [review]. Crit Care Med 2006;34(11 Suppl):S306–S308.
9. Sara M, Sacco S, Cipolla F, et al. An unexpected recovery from permanent vegetative state. Brain Inj 2007;21:101–103.
10. http:// www.nationalenquirer.com/
11. Crippen D. Medical treatment for the terminally ill: the 'risk of unacceptable badness'. Crit Care 2005;9:317–318.

Erring on the Side of Reason

Stephen Streat

I am all too familiar with the scenario described by David Crippen — a plaintive insistent request for intensive care unit (ICU) admission because "the family (or even 'the surgeon' or, much less commonly, 'the patient') want(s) everything done." This statement implies an expectation that I will admit and intensively treat the patient in the ICU.

My reaction is probably quite similar to David Crippen's reaction, that is, I focus on doing the right thing for the patient and do not feel obligated to treat the patient intensively just because someone wants it. However, the cultural, economic, moral, and legal infrastructure within which I work seems fundamentally different from that which he describes. Although some differences may seem subtle, they lead I think to very different conversations, decision making, and communication. I believe that they make it much easier for me to ensure that the right thing is done for the patient than would appear to be the case for my US colleagues.

As David Crippen points out, the concept of "futility" is peculiarly American. I suspect that it was introduced to redress what might have been seen as an unreasonable balance between what was within the bounds of reasonable possibility and the capricious and unreasonable demands of surrogate decision makers. It could then be seen as providing a higher level of moral authority for physicians' decision making, based not on full discussion of uncertainties but on mathematical certainty (or at least a level of probability which approximates it). Indeed, this point has been made by American authors[1] — "Sometimes even labeling *care* [my italics] as futile is an exercise in announcing to the family that they are now excluded from the decisionmaking process."[2]

I find the futility concept problematic — most importantly because of its meaning in common parlance of having no useful result. When used in communications with patients and families in the context of end-of-life care, it can easily be construed as implying that the physician sees "worthlessness" as a characteristic of the patient (because continuing to treat the patient is described by the physician as "futile" or "worthless"). The meaning of futility is subjective — it could be argued that any therapy that prolongs life, at any cost, has intrinsic utility; indeed some patients and families do argue this. The term is not capable of prospective operational definition and is often used imprecisely.

These deficiencies have been pointed out previously[3] but are often discounted by physicians. The absolute nature of the word is often qualified — implying that "not quite futile" is "close enough to futile" for clinical use. For example, the American Thoracic Society Guidelines on Withholding and Withdrawing Life-Sustaining Therapy[4] suggest that "...a life-sustaining intervention may be withheld or withdrawn from a patient without the consent of a patient or surrogate if the intervention is judged to be futile. A life-sustaining intervention is futile if reasoning and experience indicate that the intervention would be *highly unlikely* [my italics] to result in a meaningful survival for that patient."[5]

I contend that physicians should discuss withholding or withdrawing intensive therapies with patients and families precisely because "reasoning and experience indicate that the intervention would be highly unlikely to result in a meaningful survival for that patient," rather than because they are futile. The futility concept adds nothing to the rationale for limiting intensive therapies — rather, it is a crude device that may shift the balance of power in the discussion between physician and families while creating further opportunities for misunderstanding and distrust. We should abandon it and have the courage to speak honestly and openly with families without it.

I agree with David Crippen that physicians are not professionally obliged to treat the patient in a manner that is unreasonable, that is, not in accord with reason. However, reasonable treatment may include some active treatments, perhaps at times even some intensive treatments, as we pay simultaneous attention to comfort care — the amelioration of suffering in all its forms.[6]

Healthcare "consumers" in New Zealand have statutory rights, specified in a Code of Rights accompanying the relevant legislation[7]; the code also defines corresponding duties of healthcare providers. However, these rights do not include a right to any possible healthcare service. Not all possible services are options in the sense that the word could imply a free choice from an unlimited menu — a meaning that I think that it does easily acquire in US writings.

Consumers in New Zealand have a Right to Services of an Appropriate Standard[7] viz.

1. Every consumer has the right to have services provided with reasonable care and skill.
2. Every consumer has the right to have services provided that comply with legal, professional, ethical, and other relevant standards.
3. Every consumer has the right to have services provided in a manner consistent with his or her needs.
4. Every consumer has the right to have services provided in a manner that minimizes the potential harm to, and optimizes the quality of life of, that consumer.
5. Every consumer has the right to cooperation among providers to ensure quality and continuity of services.

The meaning of "option" is, therefore, different in New Zealand. The patient has the right to choose from services that conform to such appropriate standards — including being free to choose not to receive such services. Other options (e.g., services which are not "consistent with his or her needs") are not part of the available menu and will (usually) not be offered.

I agree that clinicians, patients, and families often focus too heavily on the chance of recovery when trying to make decisions about intensive treatments, whereas in everyday life other issues (e.g., downside risk[8]) receive equivalent attention.

Intensivists have an important leadership role in these circumstances — requiring a good understanding of post-ICU outcomes, mature communication skills, courage, compassion, and a great deal of patience. I agree with David Crippen that the subtle detail of communication with families determines the framework within which decisions are made and that physicians often lack this expertise. We should be required to obtain and maintain it.

Intensivists' expert opinions about the appropriateness of intensive treatments derives from an understanding of the clinical circumstances, the burden of treatment to the patient, the costs of treatment, the impact of treating this patient on the availability of treatment to other patients, and all the likely outcomes. All too commonly, especially when intensive treatments are used unselectively, post-ICU mortality is high — either in hospital or shortly thereafter. In addition, there is often substantial permanent decline in functional status in survivors, particularly if severe comorbidity is present or if central nervous system (CNS) damage has occurred.

Good decisions can only occur when the relevant information is both comprehensive and comprehensible. This implies that downside risk must be explicitly discussed, in simple, nonmedical terms, with appropriate opportunity for clarification and wide-ranging discussion.[9] Such discussions take time and expertise and are not suitable for delegation to a junior clinician. The substantial reported differences between family meetings in New Zealand and in the United States may be influenced by nonclinical factors (e.g., differing moral referential frameworks, organizational, and physician reimbursement practices).[10]

I agree with David Crippen that most families listen to reason, but in New Zealand they do have to as they do not have authority in the sense that competent patients have authority (or autonomy). There is no concept of surrogates by proxy and legislation does not support such a concept.

Despite the increasing use of terms such as "consumers" and "providers" in New Zealand healthcare practice,[5] intensive care services are not part of a market economy. These services are scarce and do not compete for customers who might take their business elsewhere if they aren't satisfied. Although New Zealand physicians are often reminded that poor communication is the most frequent source of complaints about treatment, there is no implication that we should just give the customers what they want.

The New Zealand media are equally lamentably facile in their reporting of anecdotal miracle awakenings. Intensivists (and our professional organizations) have a societal responsibility to bring balance to this reporting, something that we (reluctantly) do on occasion.[11]

Hospital Ethics Committees in New Zealand are seldom involved in end-of-life disputes and decision making, perhaps because of a lack of apparent need for such a role. Their role has been more to support clinicians' ethical practice. Certainly determining who are authoritative and authentic surrogates has little resonance. For example, the terms of references of my own hospitals' committee describes its purposes as:

- To provide a consultative, advisory, and supportive mechanism assisting health professionals to make their own ethical decisions (and)
- To facilitate and foster education aimed at preparing individuals to deal with ethical problems and conflicts in clinical practice.

I agree with David Crippen that some patients will die whatever treatment they receive and that they should be spared burdensome intensive treatments. When we intensivists are confronted with demands to admit and intensively treat such patients it must surely be our responsibility to instead ensure that all of their real and pressing needs (medical, psychological, emotional, and spiritual) are met.

References

1. Fins JJ, Solomon MZ. Communication in intensive care settings: the challenge of futility disputes. Crit Care Med 2001;29:N10–N1530.
2. Fins, "Communication in intensive care setting, 233.
3. Brody BA, Halevy A. Is futility a futile concept? J Med Philos 1995;20:123–144.
4. American Thoracic Society. Withholding and withdrawing life-sustaining therapy. Am Rev Res Dis 1991;144:726–731. Available at: http://www.thoracic.org/adobe/statements/withhold1-6.pdf.
5. American Thoracic Society, "Withholding and withdrawing life-sustaining therapy," 154.
6. Streat SJ. Illness trajectories are also valuable in critical care. BMJ 2005;330:1272.
7. The Health and Disability Commissioner Act 1994. Available at: http://www.hdc.org.nz/index.php.
8. Gillett G. The RUB. Risk of unacceptable badness. N Z Med J 2001;114:188–189.
9. Cassell J. Life and death in intensive care. Philadelphia: Temple University Press; 2005.
10. Streat S. When do we stop? Crit Care Resuscitation. 2005;7:227–232.
11. Let the brain damaged die, day doctors. Sydney Morning Herald. June 13, 2005. Available at: http://www.smh.com.au/news/National/Let-the-braindamaged-die-say-doctors/2005/06/12/1118514931362.html.

Healthcare Providers' Contribution to the Problem of Futility

Robert M. Arnold

Futility has become the hot topic in American bioethics as well as in intensive care units (ICUs) throughout the country. Hundreds of articles have been written defining futility and delineating the ethics of healthcare providers' unilateral decision making in futile cases; professional organizations have written position statements; hospitals have developed policies and even some states have passed legislation limiting surrogate decisions in futile situations.[1]

In the typical case of futility, the family demands unreasonable therapies that ICU providers know will not work. Despite repeated conversations, the surrogate continues to demand "everything" and biological, nonsentient life is prolonged. Because of this, families "force" their loved one to experience painful treatments prior to death. The death is undignified, the patient suffers, and scarce resources are wasted.

In this book, Crippen argues that families are given too much power to make these unreasonable choices. Family members or surrogates, he argues, do not have the expertise to make the right choices and are led astray by the popular media's focus on "miracles." Fearful of death, they grasp at mirages that only serve to prolong the dying process.[2] Streat, while agreeing that bad decisions are made, suggests that doctors talking honestly with surrogates will resolve more problems than labels such as futility. He seems to believe that the New Zealand sociopolitical environment is critical to promoting more rational conversations. The law seems to allow doctors more discretion in determining appropriate standards and thus what must be offered to surrogates in end-of-life decision making.[3] Crippen would likely argue for similar policies in the United States.

I am struck by the degree to which both of these commentaries assume that healthcare providers are victims — stuck between families who are unreasonable and a larger sociopolitical system that gives us insufficient power. What I would like to do in my commentary is discuss our responsibility for these conflicts. First, I will look at what we can do in our interactions with families to decrease requests for therapies that we do not think will work. Second, I will examine whether healthcare providers themselves have any responsibility for futile therapies. Rather than seeing healthcare providers as victims, this tack would allow us to focus on what we could do to decrease these conflicts.

Communication Skills and Futility

Why, one might ask, do surrogates, who love and care for their critically ill loved ones, demand therapies healthcare providers feel will never work? Assuming they do not want their loved ones to suffer, what rational story might one tell to explain their decision making?[4] They might not understand the biomedical situation. Empirical data suggests that when patients know the medical reality of their situation, they typically make the same choice that healthcare providers do.[5] Unfortunately, less than half of families knew what was wrong with their loved one or their prognosis 48 hours after admission to the ICU.[6]

So what could health providers do to promote understanding? First, they could meet with surrogates on a regular basis. Lilly and colleagues found that regular meetings with families decreased unnecessary treatments.[7] Yet, in the institution in which I work, regular meetings are the exception, rather than the rule. Second, we could decrease the amount of conflicting information that is provided to surrogates.[8] One way to do this is to have the same individuals meet with the family everyday. Different people are likely to present the same information slightly different, leading to misinterpretation. Another option is to decrease the number of providers who meet with the families. The opportunities for misunderstandings multiply when every subspecialist meets with the family. For example, if the nephrologist says that the kidneys are "better" and the infectious disease doctor says things are "stable," a family may not understand why the intensivist believes things are futile. Third, healthcare providers need to be more transparent, saying what they truly believe. How many times have the doctors said, "Things are grim" in rounds and then gone to the family and said they "need to keep the faith"? Moreover, families may hear qualitative predictors of prognosis (doing poorly, grim) much differently than we intend.[9] Finally, the data suggests that stress, emotions, and fatigue decrease understanding.[10] Healthcare providers need to acknowledge and attend to this psychological fact. In conversations, we could be more empathic to what the surrogate is going through. We also could develop written or computerized information that families could use to improve their understanding.[11]

A lack of information, however, may not be the only reason why family members make decisions that healthcare providers believe are unreasonable. Emotions such as guilt and sadness are often blamed for bad decision making. Here again, healthcare providers could improve the situation.

First, we could be mindful and careful about the language we use. Although never empirically studied, one can only imagine the impact of asking families if "they want us to do everything," whether we should continue to be "aggressive" or focus on "comfort care only," and whether we should "limit care." The way we talk about these decisions suggest that our goal is to do less, causing families to feel abandoned. Rather than focusing on the goals of care, we talk about stopping "life support or life sustaining therapies."[12]

Second, we could remember why we talk to surrogates — to better under-stand their loved one's goals.[13] When we say, "What do you want us to do?" the likely result is that the surrogate will feel like s/he is making a life-and-death decision. Guilt and fear are normal reactions to such a question. Given they do not want their loved one to die and they clearly do not want to feel responsible for the death, "Do everything you can" seems like the best answer. The question, "What would your loved one want, if she was sitting here and could understand what we had been talking about?" is likely to evoke a different reaction. Empirical data suggests that this question is more likely to result in the answer the patient would have given.[14] Moreover, this question is less likely to evoke feelings of guilt for the family.

Third, doctors need to be more comfortable dealing with the emotions common to end-of-life decisions. The request "do everything" may be less a statement of desire for more vasopressors and more an expression of sad-ness and frustration. The oncology literature suggests that clinicians who are uncomfortable giving bad news are more likely to offer more chemotherapy.[15] I wonder if a similar dynamic is at work in the ICU.

Finally, we need to think about the meaning of "offering" a therapy. Too often, I see doctors asking surrogates about whether they want specific thera-pies. From the family's perspective, offering a therapy may mean that it has the possibility of working. (Imagine if your mechanic asked if you wanted a new engine for your car. After you said "yes," he then spends the next 15 minutes telling you why this is the wrong decision. Wouldn't you wonder why he "offered" the choice if he did not think it was going to work?) Therapies are merely means to achieving a goal. Conversations about the goals — which ones are possible and how to achieve them — may be a way to avoid conflicts about specific therapies.

The common element among these problems is poor communication skills. A recent survey of pulmonary and critical care fellows documents scant formal teaching of communication about death and dying, little explicit feedback about basic communication skills, and an absence of role models with such expertise.[16] A separate survey of physician and nurse directors of 600 ICUs across the United States identified inadequate training and the absence of clinician–experts in communication as a major barrier to better end-of-life care of patients dying in ICUs.[17] Physicians report lacking the skills to com-municate complex medical information or to address a family's emotional needs.[18] Critical care nurses also acknowledge the inadequacy of their communication skills and training.[19]

Effective clinician–patient communication is not an inborn talent but a learned skill. Randomized, controlled trials demonstrate that brief, intensive training in communication skills significantly improves both physicians' and nurses' interviewing and counseling performances. These improvements persist following training.[20] However, I know of *no* pulmonary or critical care medicine fellowships that routinely teach and evaluate physicians' skills in this area.

Physicians' Use of Futile Therapy

Regardless of providers' communication skills, however, surrogates are sometimes going to request therapies that physicians feel are unreasonable. The question is how often this happens. The largest study on this question was the SUPPORT. They found that

of the 4301 patients, 115 (2.7%) had an estimated chance of 2-month survival of <less than or equal to> 1%. All but one of these 115 subjects died within 6 months. Almost 86% died within 5 days of prognosis. At the time of death, 92 subjects (80.0%) had had no attempt at resuscitation; 35 (30.4%) had had a life-sustaining mechanical ventilator withdrawn. A Do-Not-Resuscitate order was written either before ($n = 61$) or within 5 days ($n = 18$) of reaching this prognosis for 68.6% of the patients. These 115 subjects had total hospital charges of $8.8 million. By forgoing or withdrawing life-sustaining treatment in accord with a strict 1% futility guideline, 199 of 1688 hospital days (10.8%) would be forgone, with estimated savings of $1.2 million in hospital charges. Nearly 75% of the savings in hospital days would have resulted from stopping treatment for 12 patients, six of whom were under 51 years old, and one of whom lived 10 months.[22]

Family demands for futile care does not seem to be a large driver for medically ineffectual care. On the other hand, in the United States, the wide variations in health care suggest that physicians have some responsibility for nonbeneficial care. John Wennberg has conducted a number of studies looking at the large variations in medical care in the United States.[23] In a study of academic medical centers, he found extensive variation in the percentage of deaths associated with a stay in the intensive care (8.4%–36.8%). About a third of patients who were loyal to University of California-Los Angeles Medical Center or New York University Medical Center died in the hospital after an ICU stay, compared to 20% at University of California-San Francisco or Mount Sinai Hospital.[24] Other studies have shown wide variations in other ICU practices ranging from do not resuscitate (DNR) orders to time in the ICU prior to death.[25] Most disturbingly, these variations do not seem to correlate with better health outcomes or patient preferences.

These findings fit my personal experience. Demands for futile treatment are more likely to come from physicians than families. In my hospital, there are wide variations in physician practice. Some doctors are focused on biological life and will continue interventions to promote life even when the other healthcare providers feel that care is futile. These doctors are not interested in talking to surrogates about the patient's goals — they have decided that continued life prolonging treatment is in the patient's interest. To do otherwise, is, in their view, "playing God" or "euthanasia." These clinicians often appeal to their miracles ("I had a patient who was this sick who got better"), or their uncertainty inherent in clinical medicine ("You can not be sure he will not recover some function from that stroke over time").

If clinicians were really interested in minimizing ineffectual or futile care, they might develop policies to limit variations in their own practice. A hospital might require weekly review of all patients who met certain clinical criteria suggesting futility. They might encourage clinicians who believe their colleagues are continuing ineffectual care to speak up. For outliers, a hospital could require data from the doctor about why he believes the therapy will work. I know of no hospital that has a policy for reporting or overriding clinicians who are providing care that their colleagues believe is ineffectual.

Conclusion

A critic might point out that nothing I have suggested will stop families from requesting futile therapy. This is true and was not my goal. My goal was to decrease the *overall* frequency of ineffectual care in the ICU, regardless of who asks for it. I believe that healthcare providers have more power to decrease this care than they often admit (even in the United States). By focusing on our practices and our communication skills, I believe that we can minimize the use of futile therapies in the population of ICU patients that will die no matter what treatment is rendered them. The ball is in our court.

References

1. Fine RL. The Texas Advance Directives Act of 1999: politics and reality. HEC Forum 2001;13:59–81.
2. Crippen D. Dealing with difficult surrogates: erring on the side of autonomy. In: Crippen D, ed. End-of-life communication in the intensive care unit [this volume]. New York: Springer; 2008.
3. Streat S. Dealing with difficult surrogates: erring on the side of reason. In: Crippen D, ed. End-of-life communication in the intensive care unit [this volume]. New York: Springer; 2008.
4. Goold S, Williams B, Arnold RM. Conflicts around decisions to limit treatment: a differential diagnosis. JAMA 2000;283:909–914.
5. Weeks JC, Cook EF, O'Day SJ, et al. Relationship between cancer patients' predictions of prognosis and their treatment preferences [see comments] [published erratum appears in JAMA 2000 Jan 12;283:203]. JAMA 1998;279:1709–1714.
6. Azoulay E, Chevret S, Leleu G, et al. Half the families of intensive care unit patients experience inadequate communication with physicians. Crit Care Med 2000;28:3044–3049.
7. Lilly CM, De Meo DL, Sonna LA, et al. An intensive communication intervention for the critically ill. Am J Med 2000;109:469–475.
8. Azoulay E, Pochard F. Communication with family members of patients dying in the ICU. Curr Opin Crit Care 2003;9:545–550.
9. Chaitin E, Arnold RM. Communication in the ICU: Holding a family meeting. I and II. In: Rose B, ed. Boston: Uptodate; 2003:11.2. Revised 2005.
10. Pochard F, Azoulay E, Chevret S, et al. Symptoms of anxiety and depression in family members of intensive care unit patients: ethical hypothesis regarding decision-making capacity. Crit Care Med 2001;29:1893–1897.
11. Azoulay E, Pochard F, Chevret S, et al. Impact of a family information leaflet on effectiveness of information provided to family members of intensive care unit

patients. A multicenter, prospective, randomized, controlled trial. Am J Respir Crit Care Med 2002;165:438–442.

12. Coulehan J. I treat all my patients aggressively. J Med Humanities1990;11:193–199.
13. Buchanan AE, Brock DW. Deciding for others. Cambridge: Cambridge University Press; 1989.
14. Tomlinson T, et al. An empirical study of proxy consent for elderly persons. Gerontologist 1990;30:54–64.
15. Emanuel Z. Preliminary results on ASCO end-of-life (EOL) survey. Paper presented at: American Society of Clinical Oncology (ASCO) meeting. May 16–19, 1998.
16. Prendergast TJ, Sullivan A, Arnold RM, et al. Fellowship education in end-of-life care. Am J Respir Crit Care Med 2002;165:B4.
17. Nelson J, Cook D, Angus D, et al. End-of-life care: a survey of ICU Directors. Abstract accepted to American Thoracic Society 2003 International Conference.
18. Levy MM. End-of-life care in the intensive care unit: can we do better? Crit Care Med 2001;29:N56–N61.
19. Puntillo KA, Benner P, Drought T, et al. End-of-life issues in intensive care units: a national random survey of nurses' knowledge and beliefs. Am J Crit Care 2001;10:216–229.
20. Fallowfield L, Jenkins V, Farewell V, et al. Efficacy of a cancer research UK communication skills training model for oncologists: a randomized controlled trial. Lancet 2002;359:650–656.
21. Teno JM, Murphy D, Lynn J, et al. Prognosis-based futility guidelines: does anyone win? SUPPORT Investigators. Study to Understand Prognoses and Preferences for Outcomes and Risks of Treatment. J Am Geriatr Soc 1994;42:1202–1207.
22. Teno et al., "Prognosis-based futility guidelines," 201.
23. Wennberg JE, Fisher ES, Stukel TA, et al. Use of hospitals, physician visits, and hospice care during last six months of life among cohorts loyal to highly respected hospitals in the United States. BMJ 2004;328:607.
24. http://www.dartmouthatlas.org/. Accessed on November 20, 2005.
25. Sprung CL, Cohen SL, Sjokvist P, et al. End-of-life practices in European intensive care units: the Ethicus Study. JAMA 2003;290:790–797.

8
Emotions in the Intensive Care Unit

Ilene L. Dillon

Emotions are Part of Everything

Intensive care unit (ICU) personnel are primarily focused on the physical survival or demise of their patients. For matters of emotion and religion or belief, specialists are called in. Yet patients and their families do not compartmentalize so neatly, saving their emotional or spiritual issues for the appearance of such specialists. Emotions are a part of everything. They do, in fact, operate as guides for living (and dying), and should be a most integral part of the operation of every ICU. For purposes of discussion, we will break the areas of strongest emotion apart. In reality, emotions of patient, family, ICU doctors, nurses, and other personnel all occur simultaneously, interacting in subtle yet powerful ways. Facilitating the easy flow and validation of emotions can allow patients and families, as well as medical personnel, to accomplish their respective jobs in the ICU in the best possible manner.

Focus of Medical Personnel

In current practice, Western medicine personnel in the ICU are almost exclusively focused on the survival and/or nonsurvival of their patients. With great sophistication and information on the minute physiological changes occurring in the bodies of their charges, the medical team of the ICU focuses on making their best effort to assure the physical survival of the patient. The doctor and nurse also have the responsibility of communicating medical information to the family, including dealing with issues of possible or impending death.

Focus of Patient's Family

With a member of their family at the brink of death, the family can be seen as being in a state of crisis. Also concerned with the survival or nonsurvival of the patient, families are dealing with a huge burden of emotions. As we know, families have characteristic ways of dealing with both crisis and emotions.

These patterns are usually magnified in such a highly stressful circumstance, assuring that a family that gets angry will be angrier, one that is very loving will focus on being even more loving, and one that lives in denial, rebellion, delinquency, or repression will exaggerate these patterns.

While doctors and their ICU staff may not view identifying and dealing with the family's emotional patterns as a vital part of their job, helping families to move through their emotions can bring many positive results, such as low-ered tension and agitation, better outcome for the patient, easier interactions with hospital staff, and less likelihood of malpractice lawsuits. Five types of communication systems utilized by families have been identified.[1] Having at least a rudimentary idea of these systems can assist medical personnel in dealing more effectively with the emotional responses of the families of ICU patients. These include:

1. **The Uproar Family System** is characterized by an infantile quality, where members of the family expect loss or attack if they reveal their vulnerable, deep feelings, and thus allow barely in-control, negative contact only. A subtype of this system is the **Placater–Blamer Family System**, where some-one is always under attack and another person is always trying to make peace, a system that allows people to make contact when they otherwise could not. Approximately 30% of American families fall into the **Uproar** category.
2. **The Depressed Family System** is characterized by heaviness and deadness, accompanied by a message of hopelessness, helplessness, and guilt. There is a strong tendency to at least insinuate that others cause current difficulties, most notably by the treatment of the ICU doctor or staff. Family members tend to be self-destructive and can easily draw medical personnel into pro-tecting and working hard on behalf of the family members. Just over 10% of American families are **Depressed**.
3. **The Schizophrenic Family System** is characterized by disorganization and lack of clarity, with no one knowing where she or he stands, and decisions made only when a person feels cornered. Family members do not back up their feelings with action, and when they do act, it is out of panic or frustra-tion. Just under 10% of American families are **Schizophrenic**.
4. **The Repressive Family System** is characterized by a judgmental structure and an unwritten "rule" that "we must all be the same." Members of the family attempt to match themselves to an external, "Leave It To Beaver All American Family" image, even though there is frequently lots of just-under-the-surface anger within the family. Approximately 50% of American families are **Repressive**.
5. **The Leveling Family System** is characterized by balance, easy problem solving, clear communication, loving communications, and a willingness to face facts and work together to achieve a desired outcome. Approximately half of 1% of American families are **Leveling**.

Family systems are very strong. The primary challenge for anyone working with, or attempting communication with, families at times of peak emotion and crisis is remaining separate from the family's particular emotional system, thus enabling greater effectiveness from the medical or helping person. Many families also attempt to control and manipulate to gain whatever it is they deem necessary or important. While medical procedure protects personnel against much of this, it is still important to stay very focused, have (and follow) policy at all times, and to be willing to step away momentarily, rather than feel the surge of anger that can so easily arise when someone is attempting to manipulate!

Each of these systems facilitates or hampers the ability to face facts, as well. Unless one is working with a **Leveling Family System**, families need to be given optimal amounts of time to absorb medical and status change information, especially if they are required to make difficult life-and-death decisions regarding someone they love or to whom they feel attached.

The less emotional baggage families and family members bring to the situation, the more easily they can turn loose and allow their loved one to die. In addition to the normal processes of denial and healthy denial that are part of grief or sudden traumatic injury/illness, unresolved guilt, shame, anger, rage, unfilled needs for unconditional love, and a number of other pieces of "unfinished emotional business" cause people to hold on to family members, selfishly insisting "I'm not ready for him or her to die," rather than being able to be supportive of what is (or needs to be) happening.

ICU personnel are not therapists and cannot attend to all the emotional nuances. Yet to have an ongoing awareness and understanding of why people respond as they do can allow ICU personnel to employ more effective interventions, thus easing their job, the patient's situation, the family's stress, and the possibility of malpractice backlash.

ICU Doctors, Personnel, and Staff Emotions

We're all human. With all of our experience, training and intention to remain neutral and focus on the task at hand, human emotions are still bound to arise in regard to particular patients, families, or situations.

The ideal situation is that all ICU people have worked on themselves to the point that they are emotionally balanced at all times, able to be empathetic and compassionate while not losing boundaries or compromising their medical effectiveness, in addition to being able to allow currently arising emotions to pass through without leaving residual that could lead to taking the job home, depression, or burnout.

Medical personnel are usually expected to deal with the highly emotional human dramas encountered through intensivist medicine in the best way they can, without built-in mechanisms and procedures for processing and healing upsets, sadness, grief, anger, or rage. Much of the emotion for those working under doctors may be generated because personnel are expected to (and need to) follow directives made by others with which they may not agree. Take the case of an ICU nurse on a burn unit who worked in the Midwest. As she cared for people suffering third-degree burns over most of their bodies, she was expected to use 20 or more units of blood in an effort to save someone that medical experience indicated didn't have a chance of living. "Why waste these resources on this individual," she questioned herself, "when others who have a chance of living would derive more benefit from these units of blood?" She reports a strong internal struggle to remain focused and compassionate with the ICU patient, while following directives with which she didn't agree and which went against her own philosophy. It takes a very dedicated professional to continue acting as an effective member of the medical team in the face of this type of internal conflict, and especially to keep his or her emotional attitude from bleeding through and thus affecting staff, family, or patient status. Doctors leading ICU and trauma teams could well model on industry experts, who learned that corporate change initiated from the top of the organization required a personal buy-in from lower-level employees in order to avoid sabotage and noncompliance with the changes.

How We Educate People to Deal with Emotions

Few people, including psychotherapists of all types, understand the true nature and purpose of emotions. Through recent research and mind–body investigations, we are beginning to understand that emotional centers exist all over our bodies, and can result from or lead to chemical changes in the body.[2] We are also coming to view emotions as tools, designed to alert us to needed change or direct our actions, much as pain alerts the body to the need for attention and healing.

Most people divide emotions into "positive" and "negative," thus identifying some emotions as desirable and judging others as most undesirable. In fact, emotions are part of humans from before birth, are neutral in nature, and become "negative," only when they are stored or held onto. All emotions, held inside, grow.

Just as a river across a dam is more likely to burst during a large storm, so emotions long-held inside of people are likely to burst out during times of crisis and intensity. This means that ICU personnel are more likely to be the target of inappropriately dumped anger, rage, blame, and attacking words. Not only do such personnel need to be equipped with techniques for turning this energy aside, they also need mechanisms for releasing their emotional residual, in order to avoid negative consequences.

This is relevant in the ICU because the tendency of most people — families and ICU personnel included — is to attempt to ignore emotions, set them aside, judge particular emotions as "wrong," and work to "forget" or "get rid of" whatever emotion seems problematic at the time. All of these are futile efforts. Emotions are energy, and as such, do not disappear. They channel underground for a time, change form, or sit and grow in power. A healthier way to deal with emotions that allows their energy to move through and out of the way is to acknowledge, work with and release whatever emotions arise, utilizing them as the tools they are meant to be. Allowing emotions to pass through (medical personnel, families, patients) leaves a clean emotional atmosphere, just as a rain leaves our air smelling "fresh." The more doctors, nurses, and ICU staff can facilitate the movement of emotions (for themselves, patients, and families), the lighter the load for all. If ICU staff cannot accomplish this in addition to their physical care duties, they will benefit from understanding the importance of enlisting consultation from necessary specialists and routinely requesting their assistance.

The Intensive Care Unit Patient and Emotions

Especially because we have not had uniform and clear ways of teaching people about emotions and how to deal with them effectively, every single ICU patient will have his or her unique relationship to emotions. As we know, this means that whether they recover or die, their emotional process will have some similarities to those of others, and many distinct features as well. Whether a patient has had opportunity to digest his/her medical condition or suffered sudden onset or injury also will affect their emotional progression during their stay in the ICU. To complicate matters further, especially in our understanding of what is happening with patients emotionally, most are unconscious and also treated with a variety of drugs, many of which alter both consciousness and affect.

If a patient is advised of the medical situation ahead of time, they will proceed through the steps of grief: disbelief, bargaining, sadness, anger, acceptance, and rebuilding. Such a patient will be at whatever point in this process time has allowed. We can anticipate that such a patient will continue "processing" the information, even if on a subconscious level, because once the mind starts creating emotional change, it tends to proceed to completion.

If the injury, illness, or physical insult that lands a patient in the ICU was of sudden onset, and they are in natural or drug-induced coma, there is little way we can determine their emotional state or progress. From reports rendered by patients who have recovered, we know that some level of processing proceeds, though it is not by any means logical, orderly, or directed by the conscious mind. What we do know is that patients continue to hear and can be deeply affected by even casual comments made in their presence, thus making it vitally important for ICU personnel to take extreme care with their words while within hearing distance of a patient. Certainly if, as research has shown, a patient's mortality can be caused by a pronouncement of the doctor that s/he has an incurable illness (and spontaneous healing can occur if told of health, even while suffering an incurable illness),[3] similar effects can be assumed when a patient lies in a coma and no longer has the conscious brain to monitor and evaluate incoming communications.

Intensive Care Unit Patients and Psychosis

The question can be asked whether, and if so at what point, a dying ICU patient enters a state of psychosis. Do all dying ICU patients eventually enter a state of psychosis prior to death?

The armchair definition of *psychosis* is "out of contact with reality." If we take this as our measure of psychosis, then we could label an emotionally upset person, a small child, or even a sleeping person as psychotic. Similarly, as ICU patients fall into deeper and deeper comas or move in and out of drug-induced sleep, we could label their state as psychotic. When, exactly, they move into or out of such a psychosis would be very difficult, if not impossible, to determine.

Another interesting armchair philosophy is that "tigers don't change their stripes." As a psychotherapist with over 40 years of experience with a variety of individuals, this writer can attest that as people near natural death, they reveal more and more of their real personality. After all, when you are leaving this earth, you don't have so much to lose if you allow yourself to be the real you. Accordingly, a person who has been logical and methodical for a lifetime is not likely to suddenly (absent medical causation) become illogical and sloppy. Nor is a sane, nonpsychotic person likely to become psychotic.

In my experience, however, people who are working directly with the dying often discount the internal experience of the dying person, judging him or her on in-the-world standards, rather than on in-the-process-of-leaving-this-life standards. Allow me to give a simple example from my own experience.

Helen was almost 96. She had been a well-respected legal secretary for many years, and loved words, conversation, and intellectual discourse, along with classical music. What she most feared was going into a nursing home. After a series of small strokes, the family was obliged to place her in a nursing home. As part of her family, we visited frequently. Increasingly, the nursing staff informed us "she's really out of it today," as we arrived for our visits.

One day I arrived at the home to find Helen tied into her wheelchair, head drooping, parked in the hallway. The nurse shook his head as I walked up and stood in front of Helen, affirming "she's really out of it today." As the nurse walked away I sat down in a chair opposite Helen and said, "Well, Helen, I see you've decided to die; is that right?"

No movement. Two full minutes passed, during which she slowly lifted her head and worked to focus her eyes through the thick lenses she had been wearing since cataract surgery.

"What?!" she demanded.

"I see you've decided to die. Is that right?"

She stared at me briefly and then declared, "Yes, I've decided."

Helen was one of the people who have taught me that those who are dying are engaged in the process of dying; they have already (or quickly are) losing their interest in living and in this world. If I stay in a this-world or real-world attitude, that dying patient will certainly be out of it, even seen as psychotic. However, if one goes to the trouble and walks a few steps in the patient's shoes, that individual is not out of it. Instead, such an individual is in transition, with a body and some consciousness still in this world, and a large part of consciousness somewhere else, the exact location varying according to one's beliefs.

It is up to caregivers to venture to where the patient is, if possible, in order to better understand and facilitate what is happening. Making a judgment of psychosis or nonpsychosis helps nothing, nor is there any real way to determine our accuracy.

Just as newly arriving babies can be seen as coming to the end of a long journey, which they started on in the mother ship Womb as a tiny speck of sperm and egg, so departing individuals can be seen as embarking on a long journey. When they are busy packing and checking details for departure, they're not interested in the concerns of the medical personnel caring for them, or in the details of this world. It is more inattention than psychosis.

The Future of Emotions in the Intensive Care Unit Setting

As we gain knowledge and understanding, we realize that emotions are an integral part of illness, injury, life, and death. More and more people are seeking to learn about the emotions that are part of each and all of us, as well as to master these emotions and make them into the tools they were designed to be for us.

The intensity, medical necessity, actions of drugs, dysfunctional family systems, pain, and unconsciousness that characterize people, conditions, and patients in an ICU setting may preclude on-the-spot emotional work by ICU doctors and medical personnel. However, as we move into the more conscious future people are beginning to envision and create, emotions are destined to play an increasingly important role. Forward-thinking directors of ICU units and personnel will be well served to think about, plan for, learn about, and work with emotional states in themselves, patient families, and the patients themselves, leading inevitably to fewer legal malpractice actions, less burdened staff, and greater ease in transition.

References

1. Luthman S. Dynamic family. Palo Alto, CA: Science and Behavior Books; 1974:42–43.
2. Pert C. Molecules of emotion: the science behind mind-body medicine. New York: Touchstone; 1999.
3. Siegel B. Love, medicine and miracles: lessons learned about self-healing from a surgeon's experience with exceptional patients. New York: HarperCollins; 1988.

9
The Role of Ethics Committees in End-of-Life Care

Dan R. Thompson

In order to understand the role of the ethics committee in end-of-life (EOL) care, one needs to understand where they came from and what and who they are and are not.[1] Ethics committees came about as the result of a history of scarce resources such as transplants and dialysis, suggestions or mandates from the court, such as in the Quinlan case, state or national regulations, and the Joint Commission on Accreditation of Healthcare Organizations (JCAHO). The President's Commission for the Study of Ethical Problems in Medicine also recommended the formation of Ethics Committees.[2] Outside of the United States, they may have very different history and responsibilities and may have, as they do in the United States, very different capabilities and responsibilities. They may serve many purposes. It is important to understand what they are not. They are not the medical morals committee, the institutional review board that reviews research, or the "Baby Doe" committee (the committee that makes decisions about impaired infants).

Ethics committees are like most hospital committees. They may be institutional committees, committees of the board of trustees, committees of the administration, committees of the medical staff, or, less likely, committees of nursing or pastoral care. Having the committee emanate from a body that has the respect of all of the professional staff members will help add authority or respect for the committee. They have different authority and their opinions are frequently advisory in nature. Kelly comments about ethics committees:

Ethics committees do not make hospitals ethical. They do not have automatic expertise about ethics, just because they have the title. Some of them are excellent, some good, some fair, some worthless and meddlesome. That is not specific for ethics committees; it's the way committees are.[3]

What have the committees been charged with in the case of end-of-life decisions? Are they an educational body? Do they provide ethics consultation services? Do they develop policies? What is the expertise and experience of their members? There generally is a wide variability in structure, membership, and expertise. Critical care professionals are frequently members of ethics committees because ethical issues are common in the critical care environment and these professionals usually have an active interest. Physicians and nurses frequently make up half or two thirds of the committee. Generally, the other members come from a wide variety of other staff and may include community members. Ethicists may be professionals from inside the institution or from outside. There is frequently a professional on the staff who has expertise in ethics. Having the ethicist also be a professional staff member is generally helpful from the standpoint of respect. The question of having a lawyer on the committee is variable, but knowledge of the law may be frequently very important. If a lawyer is a member of the committee, then one needs to be careful that the conversations are not necessarily just between the lawyer and the ethicist. Make up of the committee may make the function and expertise for function in EOL care very different. For those of us who work in large tertiary medical centers with well-formed ethics consultation services and ethics committees that have existed for years, results may be very different from institutions that have a short history and no formal consultation process or abilities.

Most committees do have as part of their program the education of their members, their constituency and for the community. This may be very different from providing ethics consultations on a regular basis, but both functions are important. Education of nonmembers may include communication with patients and families at the end of life.

What, then can they provide at the end of life? The ethics consultant can help with many areas but in particular with advance directives and their use, questions about management of persistent vegetative state, surrogates, and general end-of-life issues. The experience of many routinely performing ethics consultations is similar: the question asked is frequently not the question for which the answer is sought. Also the issue is commonly not an ethics issue but frequently a communication issue. The committee may have the expertise to facilitate communication and they may be able to provide conflict resolution or mediation. Having a third party to help be the go-between for the parties frequently smoothes out communications and quiets emotions. The consultant may be able offer suggestions that can break stalemates and make it unnecessary to resort to outside help, including the legal system. However, at times the question cannot be answered. Controversy about such things as futility,[4] religious questions[5,6] and conflicts with the law frequently cannot be changed, but knowledge and understanding of the issues may be helpful in finding a compromise. Accepting of the issues may be the solution. It is important to know if there is a time limit for help and if questions answered by the on-call person or if the whole committee needs to meet.

One of the controversial issues that healthcare providers face of particular importance in the United States is the issue of autonomy. The word has its foundation in the Greek *auto* (self) and *nomy* (to govern). This refers to self-rule, determining one's own course or self-governance. Autonomy in the US culture is an important right that has its roots in legal cases and in ethical norms. The assumption is that a person that has capacity to make their own decisions and should be allowed to make their own decisions. From the healthcare provider's position, respect for autonomy is the same as respect for the patient as a person. The legal right in this aspect has been particularly reaffirmed is the legal right to refuse treatment. The right to a specific treatment does not have the same legal or ethical right, but certainly the issue of right to appropriate care is clearly supported. One of the frequent questions for ethics committees comes when there is a dispute between healthcare providers and the patient or the patient's family about the provision of therapy that one or the other to be finds futile or inappropriate and the other finds important or even mandatory.

The concept of autonomy implies that the individual has the capacity to make a rational decision, but has an understanding of the choices and options and the freedom to make such a choice. Ethics consultations are frequently about the issue of capacity, but this is not the whole answer. Capacity is task specific and a patient that cannot do one task, such as balancing their checkbook, may have the capacity to determine their own care plan. Who should determine capacity? Most appropriately it is the physician that normally cares for the patient and knows them. There is a long history of interaction and a sympathetic understanding of the patient and usually the patient has a long history of trust in such a person. Outside physicians, such as a neurologist and a psychiatrist, are the ones that do help determine competency, but they are not necessarily the best ones for determining capacity.[7,8]

The patient with capacity must have an understanding of the choices and options in their own care. Communication of between the care team and the patient should be ongoing and freely exchanged. One must remember the difference in understanding that the two individuals by nature may have. If the patient is a layperson who has a limited understanding of the process, the communication must of necessity be different from the patient who is a medical professional. At times the communication may be strained and a third party may be the better person to assist with the process. This may be a family member, friend, social worker, or, in some cases, an ethics consultant. Most consultants would rather that the routine process be by one of the former people, at least in the beginning.

The freedom of choice may be very easy or may be difficult. Is there a choice and is it obtainable? Most of the time, the treatment of the patient should, particularly in the intensive care unit or intensive therapy unit (ICU/ITU), be goal driven. Having specific goals rather than discussing specific therapies may make for a cleaner and more honest discussion. This can eliminate discussion of goals that are not obtainable or possible and at least make goals more fittingly manageable. Provision of therapy that cannot meet the specific goal can be discussed and clarified before beginning. In the ICU/ITU, the provision of therapy should be considered a trial in many cases. This implies that it may not have as a result the agreed upon goal, but rather needs to be tried to see if the goal can be reached. In the event that it does not work, the ineffectual process can be discontinued when this is determined. In reality, this upfront discussion is frequently not the case, which may lead to problems later when the discussion becomes one of stopping ineffectual therapy.

For patients in the ICU/ITU, communication may be problematic. If the patient is not sedated and intubated, then an actual conversation can begin. More likely the conversation has not occurred and the patient is either sedated and cannot be totally awakened or the patient is difficult to communicate with, as they cannot physically speak because of the presence of an endotracheal tube or tracheotomy tube. Communication with the patient who is awake still can happen, but it is much more difficult. Most intensive care physicians know how to communicate in this situation, albeit with difficulty. If no communication has occurred in the past then this is an awesome experience. Communication itself is difficult, but determining whether there is an understanding can be even more difficult, but not impossible.

The patient who is not awake is an entirely different issue. In this case we usually depend on existing documents of previous conversation whether they are in the form of documents in the various medical records or in more formal documents. The living will, advanced directive, appointment of a proxy or surrogate, or power of attorney may be the form of such a document. For the purposes of this chapter, the word *surrogate* will be used for the person so appointed.

Frequently, the document will describe the situations where the patient gives specific instructions for what they wish to be done. These documents also frequently have an if/then clause. If a certain situation happens then do or do not do these things. The if/then matter is the important issue. Understanding clearly what the patient means in this situation is the first step in understanding what is done next. Just because the patient has such a document does not routinely mean that they do not wish to be resuscitated in every situation.

The appointment of someone else to speak for a patient may be the most important issue. The document can give this person the unlimited authority to speak for the patient or may limit the choices that the individual may have. Understanding of these choices and these documents is important and a member of the ethics team can help because they usually have experience with such documents. They may provide help with the issue of discussion of care goals and limitations.

Frequently, the patient cannot take part in his or her own care, and there is no appointed person to speak for them. In this case we generally speak with family members. At times the communication is not only with the patient but also with the family. At times the patient and the family will not have the same goals and there may even be a conflict between the two. At times the family will have no specific spokesman or may not even agree between themselves. Generally we chose the spokesman according to similar rules that govern the usual consent process for medical care. The order usually is: children with majority, parents, siblings, a distant relative, or friend. At times there is no family or friend to act in behalf of the patient. In the later case the ethics committee may be called upon to act for the patient. At least in the United States, the courts have frequently agreed that this is the most appropriate or best method.

We have been assuming all along that communication has been happening and both sides are speaking and the conversation is civil. This is not always the case. There may be conflict at any stage of the process. The writer has had experience with difficulties with all parties involved in the process. There may be conflict between members of the medical team, between the medical team and the patient or surrogate, or between members of the family and surrogate. Managing these conflicts in the long run is in the best interest of all parties, but in particular in the best interest of the patient.

The critical care team and the other parties can be quite exasperated if the communication has not been happening or the miscommunications result in requests for therapy that might not be in the best interest of the patient or fit the goal or even have a possible positive benefit. One of the problems in these cases is who best speaks for the patient. While caregivers should be functioning from the position of beneficence, preventing harm, going good, and promoting the welfare of the patient, it is not always apparent that this is happening, particularly to the surrogate.[9] This does not imply that the surrogate always has an understanding of the patient's best interest or that their understanding is always correct. The advent of the Internet, popular press, television, and friends has changed some of the views that patients and surrogates can have of the process. For instance, on television shows, cardiopulmonary resuscitation (CPR) generally succeeds and the patient always recovers in minutes and is always intact. This may create unreal expectations. Patients may demand therapy that is inappropriate medically or at least unrealistic.

This may result in a conflict that makes the provision of medical care difficult. Where does the ethics consultation fit into this situation? While the understanding that the patient with capacity has the right to refuse any or all treatment, this autonomy does not necessarily give the same autonomous person the right to demand inappropriate therapy. The difference can be crucial. In the first instance, we usually honor the patient's wishes when they are similar to those of the care team. When they do not then this is more problematic and we require more proof or understanding. When the patient's or surrogate's request are clearly not similar to the treatment team then a conflict occurs. At these times if early discussion cannot resolve the issue, then consultation with an outsider that can remain neutral and has skills in conflict resolution or mediation is appropriate. Conflict resolution implies that one side usually wins and mediation may mean that there is something in the middle. In most cases in conflicts in appropriate care, mediation is the better method. These skills may or may not reside in the ethics consultant. If the person or the committee has these skills, then the results may have more satisfying result for all parties. Mediation is a skill not only for the ethics consultant, but also for the critical team.[10] Improvement of the skills of both may make the resolution of such conflict better for the patient. In Western thought we have not actively considered the notion of rationing of care, but in some small areas this has been done. Knowing that society has not usually done this, one then must question the utility of individual practitioners deciding that this is their job.

We must also remember the history of the ethics committee: specifically in the past the rationing job for scarce resources in the case of limited therapy in organ donation and dialysis. For the most part ethics committees have not been given this job at present. Social utility of care, while important, frequently does not have a place in discussion of individual therapy.

Getting results from an ethics consultation is no different than obtaining a good consultation from any other consultant. Tell that person what you want to know and give them the relevant information. What is the ethical question? Is there one? Is there a question about the living will or healthcare proxy or surrogate? How can they help? Identifying the problem is a major step in the process. Remember that physicians and nurses have responsibilities and the consultant should not be expected to do things that professionals can and should do and these should be done before the ethics consultation. On the other hand, the consultant may be able to accomplish certain things as a neutral party that the team is not able to accomplish. The skill and tools that the committee members or consultant has will vary and one should know what these are and their limitations, if any. The ethics consultant needs information also, and then generally need to be able to speak with all of the parties. Having important people be available to speak with the consultant is of major importance in starting the process.

Depending on the individual institution, who can call for an ethics consultation is important. If the person asking for the consultation is not the attending physician, notifying the attending physician is important. Generally it is not appropriate to have the attending physician veto the consultation process, but they should at least know that it is happening. Sometimes the person that asks for consultation may wish to have their identity kept in confidence. While this can be understandable, it also can be problematic. Families and patients also need to know of the process and perhaps even how to ask for consultation.

At times the important issue is being able to have a face-to-face meeting and the consultation staff person can facilitate this. That person should be one that at least has the appearance to having no conflict of interest. At times it also may be important for the face-to-face meeting to include the whole committee, but this is usually not necessary. The meeting will be a time for both sides to discuss the situation and understand the other position and possibly have a dialogue. The consultant can work on mediating the situation. At times the consultant will not be able to change things, but will be only be able to start a dialogue that can result in trust and perhaps in future change.

The ethics consultant can answer questions, provide mediation and conflict resolution, and provide support for family and professional staff. At times people just need to know that they are doing the right thing. Sometimes it is a matter of knowing the right thing and this may involve understanding of the law and religious and ethical issues. Sometimes it is important for all involved to know that others share their opinion. At times it is a matter of trying to work on bringing understanding. This may require several meetings.

Where will ethics committees be in the future? A more professional role and ability should be the goal of every committee. This may not only be in the committee itself, but also in the educational work that they should and do provide. The committee should also do self-assessment of what they do and assessment of the needs of the institution and local areas that they serve. The area of ethics consultation is expanding and there are opportunities for further education for all those involved.[1]

Doing a little homework before asking for the consultation may make things easier and the results more useful.

- Know the abilities and the limitations of the specific ethics committee you are consulting.
- Tell the person who comes to start the ethics consultation what you want to know in as specific terms as possible.
- Provide them with as much information as is possible.
- Be sure that the question that you want answered is really something that can be answered.
- Remember that the consultant or committee can be a good support mechanism for staff and family members who are suffering stress about some particular ethical issue.

References

1. Thompson DR, Kummer HB, eds. Critical care ethics: a practice guide from the ACCM ethics committee. Des Plaines, IL: Society of Critical Care Medicine; 2005.
2. Jonsen AR, Siegler M, Winslade WJ. Clinical ethics — a practical approach to ethical decisions in clinical medicine. 5th ed. New York: McGraw-Hill Medical Publishing; 2002.
3. Kelly DF. Critical care ethics: treatment decisions in American hospitals. Kansas City, MO: Sheed & Ward; 1991:156.
4. The Ethics Committee of the Society of Critical Care Medicine. Consensus statement of the SCCM Ethics Committee regarding futile and other possible inadvisable treatments. Crit Care Med 1997;25:887–891.
5. Mackler A, ed. Introduction to Jewish and Catholic bioethics. Washington, DC: Georgetown University Press; 2003.
6. Kelly DF. Contemporary Catholic health care ethics. Washington, DC: Georgetown University Press; 2004.
7. Grisso T, Appelbaum PS. Assessing competence to consent to treatment: a guide for physicians and other health professionals. New York: Oxford University Press; 1996.
8. Berg JW, Appelbaum PS, Lidz CW, Parker LS. Informed consent, legal theory and clinical practice. 2nd ed. Oxford: Oxford University Press; 2001.
9. Beauchamp T, Childress J. Principles of biomedical ethics. 5th ed. Oxford: Oxford University Press; 2001.
10. Dubler NN, Liebman CB. Bioethics mediation: a guide to shaping shared solutions. New York: United Hospital Fund of New York; 2004.

10
Medical Liability Issues in Dealing with Critical Care Patients in the End-of-Life Situation

Robert A. Fink

As with almost all issues of medical liability, it is *communication* that is the critical factor in determining whether something a medical professional does or omits doing will result in a medical malpractice action. While good communication between physician and other health professionals and patients/families will not guarantee a total absence of lawsuits, poor communication, especially if associated with a less-than-optimal case outcome, will almost assuredly bring the workings of the medical tort system upon one's head. Such communication involves not only that between the physician and patient (if the critical care patient is mentally competent), but also between all involved health professionals and the extended family of the patient, including not only relatives, but, in some cases, friends and other significant others. Just think of the long-lost relative who, in a preterminal situation, arrives and, by external influence, upsets the proverbial applecart of rapport between health professionals and patient/family, and converts a calm and sensitive situation into sheer chaos — and possibly, a visit to the attorney's office.

Patients and families usually sue health professionals not because of medical damages, but rather because they want to *punish* the professional for a less-than-optimal outcome. When good communication exists between professionals and families, the urge to punish is strongly diminished (who would anyone want to punish a friend who was trying to do his/her best for a family member?), and concomitantly, when good communication has resulted in true informed consent and patient/family education, families will not be faced with sudden "surprises" and unexpected loss. When patients/families sue doctors, they usually do so to gain "revenge" for some perceived transgression on the part of the treating personnel, whether this alleged transgression is real or imagined.

The doctor who is of borderline technical competence but who has a good emotional rapport with a patient/family is not going to be sued as often, even in the presence of a poor outcome, than is the more competent physician who is perceived as "detached," uncaring, or otherwise unreachable or "cold." I have known some doctors who had such powerful rapport with their patients that had those physicians recommended a procedure such as a decapitation, the response might have been, "Sure, doc, anything you say ..."

Not only is it consonant with the traditional art of medicine to develop a good rapport with patients and families, but also it is the first line of defense against becoming involved in a legal action challenging your management of a patient. In the critical care situation, and especially, in an end-of-life context, such rapport should be secondary only to actual medical competence in the diagnosis and treatment of patients.

Communication issues can, and often do, serve as the actual trigger to a malpractice action. Years ago, our hospital was the subject by a political attack by the radical political elements in our area, and a gigantic protest was mounted, which included hearings that were held by the city council. It was alleged that our hospital did not provide humane treatment to our patients and the protest was designed to block a much-needed expansion plan for the facility's emergency department.

At the hearing (and I was one of the people who was asked to speak for the hospital), an elderly woman, who had also just filed a malpractice suit against the hospital over her experience in the emergency department, approached the microphone and related how the hospital had inflicted "torture" upon her by "keeping (her) in the emergency department for hours without feeding (her)." Furthermore, they "stuck a tube in my nose and wouldn't let me get out of bed...." I asked the patient what her diagnosis had been and she responded, "I had a bleeding ulcer," and it was obvious that she had ultimately gotten a good result from treatment. However, it certainly was apparent that no one had been particularly successful in the communications sphere and discussed with her the rationale of her (appropriate) treatment in a way that she could understand.

Think instead of a situation (such as I participated in a few years ago) in which a gunshot wound victim was being prepared for surgery (craniotomy) in the middle of the night, and the family, beside itself with grief at the impending loss of a teenager, was inconsolable and causing a near-disturbance in the emergency department. Sensing that this family was identified with a religious group (in this case, Roman Catholicism), I asked whether they wished for a priest to be summoned, and when they responded in the affirmative, I called a close friend, whose parish was only a few blocks from the hospital. As expected, he came in immediately, and was able to administer the Last Rites to the patient with the family present. In addition, the attending physician (myself), participated in the rites as well, and this "diversion" (which consumed less than 5 minutes) was all that this family needed in order to become cooperative and trusting.

Sadly, after a 3-hour operation, we were unable to reverse the major cerebral damage inflicted by the bullet, and the patient, after a brief period on life support, was declared dead and support was removed with absolutely no objection from the family. Indeed, the family members had nothing but praise for those healthcare professionals who had cared for their relative. This kind of case is replete with risk for litigation, but in this instance, there was really no way that anyone would have expected to have a litigious outcome. What was, overall, a tragic situation was converted into an experience where a grieving family had the support that it needed to carry it through a difficult event; and, at the same time, the medical providers were protecting themselves from the stresses of a malpractice suit.

Communication Involving Ancillary Personnel

While positive communication skills are important in the case of the attending physician(s), the relationship between ancillary personnel and the patients/ families may be even more critical in the prevention of malpractice allegations. Attending physicians usually spend only a few minutes each day with each patient as compared to the much greater temporal involvement in patient care provided by nurses, respiratory and other such therapists, aides, and others, who are generally employees of the hospital and not under the direct control of the attending physician. Patients who eventually leave the critical care areas and return to normal functioning almost always recall the nursing and other ancillary care with far greater intensity than the actions of the physicians, even though it may well be the latter which has resulted in the positive outcome and the saving of the patient's life.

If such ancillary personnel express negative commentary regarding the patient's care, even if such is totally unwarranted, such can become a powerful force leading towards the development of a litigious patient. This can include dissatisfaction that employees might have with the workplace, working conditions, even salary and benefits, which may have absolutely nothing to do with the quality of care that the patient is receiving. Some of these comments can be quite superficial or even innocent, such as: "Gee, that's a pretty big scar that you have…" or "Boy, Doctor XYZ took a pretty big chunk out of your bowel…" These comments, often made in ignorance of the true medical issues, may raise questions in the minds of patients and families that actually are unfounded, insignificant, untrue, and in no way indicative of any medical negligence.

The way of dealing with such personnel-introduced irritants is to foster a positive relationship between physicians and ancillary personnel and other subordinates, and, in so doing, encourage personnel to share their concerns with their superiors without fear of reprisal or criticism. A contented and appreciated staff is a powerful inhibitor of malpractice litigation.

Body Language

When patients and families are facing the loss of self or a loved one from illness or injury, there is a major impact on self-esteem. I can recall the personal experience, many years ago, when I was myself hospitalized for an infectious illness and was placed in isolation. I truly felt like the proverbial leper — an "unclean" individual who was to be feared and avoided at all costs. I immediately began to categorize my friends who came to visit me (I was in isolation for 4 days) into two groups: those who went through the hand-washing/gown/mask ritual in order to come into my room and truly visit with me; and those who opened the door, smiled, said a few superficial words, and then left without entering the room. This dichotomy has affected me to this day, some 35 years later.

During the above isolation experience, I discovered the position of subservience and infantilization that most patients with serious illness experience. One is at the mercy of others, and recovery is dependent on those over whom a patient has little or no control. I discovered, however, that one of the ways that I could assert my own sense of self-esteem was by using the electric controls of the hospital bed, to "crank up" the level of the bed so that I could approach eye level with those who came into my room, especially when I had to undergo painful or uncomfortable treatments. This "higher level" status made me feel like less of a specimen, helped me to feel more in control of what was going on, and helped to preserve my spirits during a very difficult time. So this must surely be with patients in critical care areas, and I do not doubt that their families have similar feelings at times.

Sometimes, self-therapy such as described above (the bed-raising) could be a distraction to the hospital staff, accustomed to their own routines. During the same hospitalization, I was offered the traditional bed bath (for patients who were ordered to be on bed rest), but I insisted on being allowed to bathe myself in the attached bathroom (with a nurse standing by in case of problems). This caused somewhat of a stir among the nursing personnel, but there were no mishaps and eventually all involved felt much better. Allowing patients, and by reflection, their families, as much autonomy as is possible, cultivates the quality of communication that is vital in avoiding litigation later should problems in treatment supervene.

Another bit of body language that I have discovered over the years has been related to the manner in which one presents "bad news" to patients and their families. Imagine, for a moment, a 6-foot-tall physician, weighing 200+ pounds, standing in front of a dying patient or a grief-stricken family, and somberly intoning a grave prognosis ("hanging crepe," as one of my intensivist colleagues called it). This can be an overwhelming experience for family members (and may serve as the seed for a later lawsuit to "punish" the healthcare providers). In such circumstances, I always attempt to *physically* assume an equal or slightly lower level of posture when discussing such serious issues. This may mean pulling up a chair and sitting down when conversing with the patient/family, and there have been instances, when no chairs were available, that I have actually sat down on the floor during such discussions. I have had much positive feedback from patients and families regarding this.

Communication and Personal Emotions

In medicine, traditional wisdom usually dictates that a physician should maintain detachment from his/her patients. We are told that failure to observe emotional boundaries can be detrimental to a patient, and while this can be true in some cases, such is not always the case, especially in a situation such as an impending or actual death situation. There is a tendency to forget that fact that, in some cases, a degree of attachment can be healing, both for the patient/family and the physician. I recall, at a clinical conference during which I presented an end-of-life case from the intensive care unit (ICU), and discussed my management of the last hours of the patient's life, I was strongly attacked by one of my colleagues (interestingly, a primary care physician), who accused me of "getting involved with (my) patients." I replied by saying, "Yes, I get involved with patients all the time, but only when it is helpful to the patient or the family and does not violate the basic canons of our profession."

We are all human beings, and only the most jaded and insulated among us can coldly watch a fellow human suffer and die, especially one who is doing so "before their time" or under painful circumstances. Patients and families want their physicians to be *humans*, not robots, and the demonstration of an appropriate degree of human emotion around a dying patient is something that should not be condemned. A simple hug extended to the close family of a recently deceased patient is not only a normal human response, but this all-so-human act may be a significant factor in the prevention of a malpractice suit.

Legal Issues

I have saved the discussion of the purely legal issues for the end of this chapter. This is because, in my opinion, they are the least pertinent in the avoidance of malpractice actions related to patients and families involved in end-of-life situations. Most physicians and many other healthcare providers are well imbued with the knowledge of the basic legal guidelines when it comes to the treatment of patients, and the legal system is actually relatively clear cut in such issues.

Protecting oneself from the purely legal foibles of the tort system can best be summed up by the oft-repeated and repetitive phrase: "Document, document, and document!" Charting, by physicians and ancillary personnel, should be detailed, frequent, and legible. Illegibility of chart entries is, in my experience as a reviewer of malpractice cases, one of the most destructive factors in the defense of allegations of negligence, and, among charting issues, are second only to the lack of *timing* of critical entries. Chart entries must be legible and carefully timed; if a person is handicapped by a poor handwriting, then chart entries must be dictated and transcribed, or, as in increasingly popular at many hospitals, typed on the terminals located in most nurses stations. It also suffices to say that, in the matter of charting, entries should not be altered in any way without making such alterations clearly identifiable as such, and allowing the initial entry to remain as well as the altered one. Seeing an altered note in a chart without an explanation is tantamount to a judgment for a plaintiff in a medical negligence case.

The other bit of valuable prophylaxis against legally based malpractice suits is that of the use of liberal consultation. Not only is such consultation beneficial for the patient, but also, as venerable Ben Franklin said (paraphrased) when discussing the Declaration of Independence in 1776, "We had better stand together, otherwise, we shall surely hang together ..."

Conclusion

There is no way in which one can totally insulate oneself against allegations of negligence that are made by patients and/or families. Maintaining good communication and sensitivity with patients/families, and allowing one's human characteristics to show through the professional persona are, in my view, the most effective means in which to avoid the stress, pain, and cost of legal actions. Opening oneself to one's human side is also quite effective in maintaining one's own mental health, as those of us who work with patients who are critically ill and often with end-of-life issues can be emotionally injured in ways which do not appear until later, and which can lead to delayed complications in healthcare personnel, including such entities as depression, alcohol and/or drug abuse, or even suicide.

The above principles, along with an obsessive dedication to proper documentation, will go a long way to protect medical professionals against the risks of legal challenge. This protection will extend to virtually all types of clinical situations, but in the case of critical care patients who are in extremis, the effects of this approach are even more effective.

11
End-of-Life Issues and United States Politics

Errington C. Thompson

In medical ethics, there are some things that are clearly established. Patients who are competent do have the right to participate in their own care. In 1914, Justice Cardozo wrote, "Every human being of adult years and sound mind has the right to determine what shall be done with his body."[1] This continues to be true today.

In the late 1960s and early 1970s, ventilator management was being perfected. Intensive care units (ICUs) began to crop up throughout the country. At the same time, there were advances in fluid and electrolyte management of many disease processes. New and better antibiotics were being developed. New, different, and more invasive surgical techniques were being perfected, including coronary artery bypass, organ transplantation, and aortobifemoral bypass grafting. I do not mean to insinuate that these operations were not performed on a limited basis earlier. But during this time period these therapies became more widely available. Tilney wrote one of the earliest reports of multiple organ dysfunction syndrome in 1973.[2] Multiple organ dysfunction syndrome and all of its variations pushed the medical community to do more for its patients. More intensive care. More and better ventilator management. Better management of shock. Better everything except now patients are living much longer with much more ailments. This atmosphere creates medical dilemmas that were not thought of in the 1940s and 1950s.

This brings us to the 1976 case of Karen Quinlan. Karen went to a party with her friends. She had some alcohol and some Valium. She was found sometime later apneic. This case drew international attention when Karen's parents petitioned the court to remove the ventilator against the wishes of her doctors. The New Jersey Supreme Court stated that a person has a right to refuse medical care and that this right is not lost just because the person is incompetent. A 1975 *Time* magazine article entitled the "Right to Live — or Die" stated

Karen's case raises age-old medico-legal questions about human life, now complicated by technology's ability to keep gravely injured victims at the borders of survival. Is there a point at which incurable illness becomes living death? If so, is it permissible for someone's life to be deliberately cut off? And who has the right to make such a decision?[3]

Two major movements grew out of the Karen Quinlan case. States began to institute living will legislation and hospitals began to form ethics committees to help deal with situations like this. Unfortunately, the Karen Quinlan case only set law in the state of New Jersey.[4]

The United States Supreme Court decided the next major case in 1990. Nancy Cruzan was a young woman who was involved in a motor vehicle crash. At the time the case was argued before the US Supreme Court, Miss Cruzan was not on a ventilator but was in a persistent vegetative state. A feeding tube was feeding her. The Missouri Supreme Court stated that Nancy had the right of self-determination. Because she was incompetent, the Missouri Supreme Court agreed that the parents did have the right to speak for her *but* they needed to provide clear and convincing evidence of her wishes. The US Supreme Court in a 5-to-4 decision agreed with the Missouri Supreme Court. The US Supreme Court stated that individual states could decide the level of proof needed to be provided by the surrogate who is speaking for the patient.[4] The feeding tube was removed from Nancy Cruzan.

In both of the aforementioned cases, the parents were in agreement with the course of action. There was no spouse. In a way, these cases were relatively simple because everyone who was speaking for the patient was saying the same thing.

Terri Schiavo was a 27-year-old woman who suffered a cardiac arrest in 1990. She, like Nancy Cruzan, was in a persistent vegetative state. She was not on a ventilator. Her husband (Michael) and her parents, Bob and Mary Schindler, diligently cared for her for 2 or 3 years. The relationship between the husband and her parents began to fracture around the time of a malpractice settlement dealing with Terri's 1990 cardiac arrest. The malpractice suit was settled in 1993. In 1994, Mr. Schiavo decided not to treat one of Terri's infections. What was left of any family harmony now irreparably breaks down. The parents of Terri Schiavo went to court to force the doctors to treat Terri. This is the beginning of what became an 11-year battle over the fate of Terri Schiavo.[5]

The courts consistently focused on the pertinent questions in this case. Who spoke for Terri Schiavo? Did she ever give clear and convincing evidence (the Florida statute is written much like the Missouri statute) of her wishes prior to her cardiac arrest in 1990? In 2001, a trial judge ruled that Terri Schiavo would not have wanted to live in a persistent vegetative state. The Florida court of appeals agreed with the trial judge. The Florida Supreme Court refused to hear the case.[5]

Unfortunately, this saga did not end with the Florida Supreme Court. Politicians became involved on both sides. This case was elevated from a private battle between Michael Schiavo and Bob and Mary Schindler to something much larger and much uglier. National organizations began to line up and choose sides. The Florida legislature became involved. Florida Governor Jeb Bush became involved. The ugliness began to peak when Governor Bush states, "There's this rush to starve her to death."[6]

The United States Congress entered the picture. Speaker of the House Tom Delay and Senate majority leader Bill Frist pushed for legislation to have the feeding tube permanently replaced. Senator Bill Frist, a cardiac surgeon, stated on the floor of the Senate, "I question it (persistent vegetative state) based on a review of the video footage which I spent an hour or so looking at last night in my office." He went on to say, "She certainly seems to respond to visual stimuli."[7] He stated this without examining Ms. Schiavo and in spite of the fact that four neurologists had examined Terri since 2002 and that they all came to the same conclusion: Terri Schiavo was in a persistent vegetative state.

Both the United States House and Senate passed legislation written specifically for Terri Schiavo. President George W. Bush signed the bill into law, which federalized Terri Schiavo's case and called for the feeding tube not to be removed until the federal review was complete. With unusual speed the federal courts reviewed the merits of the case and agreed with the lower courts. The United States Supreme Court refused to hear the case. Terri's feeding tube was removed and she was allowed to die.

If we step back and take an international view of the medical ethics that surround the persistent vegetative state, there really is not a clear picture. Physicians in countries like England, New Zealand, South Africa, and Brazil confront a patient like Terri Schiavo in different ways. The best example of the two extremes may be from South Africa. In a private hospital, patients in a persistent vegetative state may receive the same kind of aggressive care that Terri Schiavo got. On the other hand, in a government hospital, patients with Glasgow Coma Scales less than 10 72 hours after admission are extubated and sent to the floor (E. Hodgson, personal communication). In many countries, advanced ICU care and other tests (somatosensory evoked potentials, computed tomography scans, magnetic resonance imaging) are not available for these types of patients. England's recent court case of Miss B., who was a very high quadriplegic from a high cervical lesion, had to petition for the right of self-determination to be taken off a ventilator (N. Macartney, personal communication).

Finally, after reviewing the Terri Schiavo case, one can come away very disheartened. We, as Americans, should have been asked to do more than simply choose sides. A thoughtful discussion in state legislatures and Congress should have been generated around end-of-life issues. It is true that some Americans did fill out living wills and had frank discussions with their family members about end-of-life desires. This is a great start. We must do more. Think back to that 1975 *Time* article that was quoted earlier. Can we answer these questions yet? "Is there a point at which incurable illness becomes living death? If so, is it permissible for someone's life to be deliberately cut off? And who has the right to make such a decision?"[3] It is time for us to work with our state governments and find some answers that we all can live with. National guidelines could help lift the burden of guilt that some families feel when they withdraw therapy. We must work toward keeping these patients out of the courts. We, as physicians, nurses, and ethicists, must work toward resolving these cases at the bedside. We must work with the families through these difficult times and help them cope with a variety of emotions.

References

1. Singer PA, Siegler M. Cecil textbook of medicine. 21st ed. Philadelphia: Saunders; 2000:5.
2. Tilney NL, Bailey GL, Morgan AP. Sequential system failure after rupture of abdominal aortic aneurysms: an unsolved problem in postoperative care. Ann Surg 1973;178:117–122.
3. The right to live — or die. *Time*. October 27, 1975. Available at: http://www.time.com/time/archive/preview/0,10987,913579,00.html. Accessed January 15, 2006.
4. Annas GJ. "Culture of life" politics at the bedside. The case of Terri Schiavo. N Engl J Med 2005;352:1710–1715.
5. Quill TE. Terri Schiavo: a tragedy compounded. N Engl J Med 2005;352:1630–1633.
6. Stacy, M. Doctors remove Terri Schiavo's feeding tube after last-ditch congressional effort fails. *The Seattle Times*. March 18, 2005. Available at: http://seattletimes.nwsource.com/html/nationworld/2002211412_schiavo18.html. Accessed January 15, 2006.
7. Babington C. Viewing videotape, Frist disputes Fla. doctors' diagnosis of Schiavo. *Washington Post*. March 19, 2005:A15.

12
Comments from Ancillary Healthcare Providers

My Experiences with End-of-Life as a Bedside Nurse

Amy Seligman

I have a hunch that this chapter will be very unlike other chapters in this book. I have been a nurse for over 13 years. Seven of those years have been spent in critical care. I work in a neurovascular intensive care unit (ICU) in a major university hospital. Many times patients come to us in an obtunded state and never become fully awake during their stay. Other times their admission uncovers a life-threatening or a life-changing diagnosis and quality-of-life and end-of-life questions are staring them in the face. I have seen in my recent experience greater use of palliative care services utilizing a multidisciplinary approach with clearly defined goals and priorities. I have learned a lot from being a participant in these end-of-life discussions. They provide a forum for families to gain information and communicate their worst fears, their best hopes, and their wishes for their loved ones. However, the greatest lessons that I have learned about death have come from my patients. Often it comes at night when much of the traffic in the ICU has quieted down and the patient and their family are alone with their thoughts. I might have been just about to leave the room and click off the light and a voice calls out. As a nurse you recognize this voice and know that it is a different request than the others before it and you listen.

I had a patient. He was a physician who had recently been diagnosed with renal cell carcinoma with metastases. When I received shift report from the nurse who was leaving for the day, she commented that this particular patient was on the call bell constantly and wanted to get out of bed every hour. She said that obviously he did not need to be in an ICU anymore. She said that he was very trying.

Sure enough, before I was even out of report, I got a call from this patient. I went into his room and he wanted to get out of bed and walk the halls NOW. I explained that I was very busy and had to do my first med rounds and assessments but I would be back at 8 P.M. and take him for a walk. I have found with anxious patients that if you meet their initial requests with reliability they often calm down and begin to trust. I did return at 8 P.M. as promised and I gathered my patient's many tubes and IV poles and we began to walk. He explained to me that it was very important for him to walk as he had just made a decision not to be reintubated given his prognosis. Being a physician he was very aware of the need for good pulmonary toilet and ambulation. I told him that I understood.

I then asked him about his family. Was he married? How many children did he have? What kinds of things did they do? Where did they go to college? I exchanged information about my family. Before we knew it we were laughing about a funny family story. Then there was a long pause in our conversation. My physician patient stopped and looked at me and said, "You don't know what a pleasure it has been to have a normal conversation with someone. Ever since I have been in the hospital, I have done nothing but talk to physicians and nurses about my prognosis, possible treatment options, code status, and so on. When I look at my wife's face, I can see that she is scared to death. It paralyzes us and we can't even talk about anything. I just want to thank you for talking with me about *me* and not my disease."

It is so important to remember that just because a patient is dying it doesn't mean that he has stopped living. Take time to know your patient instead of using medicine as a shield against the pain of death.

Often we don't initially recognize that our patient is dying. We had a patient whom I'll call Marjorie. Marjorie was a woman in her 60s who had a cerebellar hemorrhage. She did very well after the neurosurgeons performed a craniotomy and clot evacuation. She was alert and following commands. She had a smoking history and developed pneumonia. She had difficulty weaning from the ventilator but she had an early tracheostomy in hopes of improving her ability to wean from the ventilator. The nurses recognized that it was important to encourage the patient to focus on her progress. We got to know her husband very well and her son. We had a communication board and let her point to pictures, letters, and words to try to communicate with us. On her birthday, we had a cake and sang to her. Days turned into months in the ICU and she developed complication after complication. Twice she did wean from the ventilator and was on a neurosurgery floor and came very close to being discharged to rehab only to be readmitted to the ICU. The last readmission that Marjorie had to the ICU involved an abrupt change in her neurological status and she was in kidney failure. On seeing her husband back in the ICU and attending a meeting with him and the critical care physicians, I noticed what a toll his wife's hospitalization was taking on him. He had obviously lost weight and his face told the tale. I talked with him and we talked about the fact that he had some hard decisions to make. The doctors were recommending dialysis or Marjorie would die. They explained that she was in multisystem failure.

After the meeting, Marjorie's husband caught me up on the events that had passed since leaving the ICU. I asked him if during one of the periods when his wife was off the ventilator and able to speak, had they talked about what she would want if things got worse? He said that they had but that she had been so close to leaving the hospital twice before that he didn't want to feel like he was giving up too soon. Marjorie was obtunded now.

Marjorie's husband wanted to talk to me about Marjorie. He told me about how the two of them had met and where they had lived when they were first married. He shared details about what her interests were before she was ill. Often when family members are faced with the loss of their loved one they will reminisce and do a sort of life review. Marjorie's husband asked if she was in pain. He asked if I thought she could hear him. He asked what it would be like if we removed life support. He asked if she would suffer. I answered his questions as I have answered these same questions hundreds of times before for families that were in this circumstance. I explained that we would make her comfortable. I said that hearing is the last to go and that he should talk to her and tell her things that he wanted to say to her. I told him that his voice and his touch would be comforting to her.

These are the things that almost every person wants to know for their dying family member. They want their loved one to know that on some level that they are there with them. They want to be assured that they are not experiencing pain or suffering and they want the people that are caring for their loved one at the end of their life to know what that person means to them. Marjorie's husband, by telling me about her life, was beginning to accept her death. He was recognizing that this would be the way in which she will continue to go on for him after her death. She will live by his stories and his memories of her. Often this life review is the practice for what the new reality will be when the patient dies.

Medicine is very aggressive and very fast paced and some times it is hard to shift gears from aggressively trying to save a life to finding the time to stay a little while longer at the bedside and hear what the patient or family member is trying to find the courage to say. Whether you are helping your dying patient to find his voice and face his fears or helping a family member of a dying patient to face the inevitable, a nurse is an important bridge. The thing that I have learned from participating in hundreds of deaths is that every death is the first time for that person and that family that are experiencing it. Nurses share in some of the most important life events of their patients and their families. When that event is death, nurses seem to know intuitively that listening is the most important thing that they can do to help the healing to begin.

A Chaplain's Perspective

Leslie Beckhart Jenal

From a chaplain's perspective, suffering is a spiritual as well as an ethical and medical phenomenon. Suffering threatens the personhood of the patient, where *personhood* is defined as having the potential to pursue fundamental values. These values include spiritual values, and personhood is accordingly itself a spiritual value. Therefore, suffering has a teleological significance; pain causes suffering because it affects the inherent pursuit of values, and hence the spiritual value of personhood.

From a spiritual and a religious perspective, suffering may have transformative or redemptive meaning for the patient, for as the ability to pursue values is limited by suffering, values may change. What seemed so important before now may seem insignificant. However, in order for suffering to be meaningful, two requirements must be met. First, the patient must have sufficient physical, intellectual, psychological, and spiritual resources to participate with God in finding meaning in suffering. A minimally responsive or unresponsive patient, or a patient without sufficient resources, does not experience meaningful suffering. Second, suffering must be necessary, that is, suffering must not be the result of medically inappropriate interventions, regardless whether those interventions are physiologically futile or not.[1] Meaningless suffering is therefore an evil. Biological life is sacred but finite; it is a nonmoral or prima facie value, but it is not an absolute value. Accordingly, death is a nonmoral or prima facie evil, but it is not an absolute evil. In point of fact, most spiritual and religious traditions hold that life after death has a greater value than this life, and certainly has a greater value than biological life. To hold biological life out as the ultimate value is to subordinate personhood, a spiritual value, to a finite value, and is, from a religious standpoint, to engage in idolatry. Therefore, the relief of suffering, even where it leads to death, may have greater value than biological life in circumstances where further medical treatment is inappropriate.

In this chapter, I will explore some of the psychological and religious reasons why, when a moribund and unresponsive or minimally responsive patient experiences meaningless suffering, and a physician has determined that further life-sustaining interventions are inappropriate, a family may resist the withdrawal of those interventions.[2] Ideally, the family will respect an advance directive in force, or a legitimate substituted judgment, although a higher evidentiary standard should be required where the burden is extreme or where the decision is unconventional.[3] From an ethical standpoint, where the patient's interest conflicts with that of the family, to concede to the family is to abandon the patient.

A patient's identity is affected, but is not constituted, by family relationships. Decisions about patient treatment will affect family relationships that survive the patient's death, and family dynamics affect decisions. Preexisting

134

rifts in the family structure are frequently exacerbated when a patient is dying, and new alliances for or against one or more family members may be made. In certain cases, family members may disagree primarily in order to thwart each other. Not infrequently, the position of a family caregiver conflicts with the position of other family members, not necessarily because further care of the patient would be burdensome to the caregiver, but often because that caregiver has a clearer vision of the patient's quality of life. A chaplain may arbitrate between the different factions and reinforce the point that the patient's interest takes precedence over unhealthy family dynamics.

Often, conflict arises because the family members need resolution with the patient even if the patient's condition makes that resolution impossible. Where the patient has abandoned his family, perhaps due to alcoholism, drug abuse, or mental illness, family members may want the love from the patient that they never received. Conversely, a family member who is estranged from the patient may refuse to give consent to withdraw life-sustaining interventions out of guilt. Family members also frequently feel guilty at not having done enough, including not caring for the patient at home or not visiting the patient often. There is rarely enough time for professional counseling to have much effect. Alternatively, family members may want the patient to stay alive in the hope that he will regain consciousness and that they can say goodbye; unfortunately, this possibility is often offered by healthcare providers.[4] Family members also may believe that not demanding every possible intervention will mean that they have abandoned the patient.[5] A chaplain will be able to discuss this belief with the family.

A family may resist medical evidence because the patient is a "fighter." This may happen where the patient's condition is chronic or long term, and the patient has survived critical, life-threatening episodes in the past. Family members frequently believe that just because the patient has survived past episodes, he will survive this one, despite all evidence to the contrary. Or, as is often the case, family members may resist medical advice because of anecdotal evidence or inaccurate information from the media.

On the other hand, physicians are sometimes responsible for a family resisting the withdrawal of life-sustaining interventions. Family members can make autonomous decisions only when they have sufficient information. A family cannot exercise autonomy by selecting from a list of all possible interventions and then being asked if they want "everything" done. Nor should a physician confuse giving hope with failure to provide accurate medical information, including an estimated prognosis, if possible. For a myriad of reasons, some family members may not understand medical information sufficiently to form questions. Chaplains can translate medical terms of art but may feel constrained lest they be seen to be providing medical advice. It may be more appropriate for a chaplain to ask obvious questions in family meetings with the physician so that information can be clarified. In addition, a family may not understand the significance of the patient's condition when he does not appear to be suffering. It is often helpful to explain what drugs are being prescribed, with special attention, for example, to sedation to enable the patient to tolerate a ventilator.

In addition, a physician's communication style may emphasize the information gap between that physician and the family, with the result that the family resists the physician's knowledge, skill, and expertise, or may intimidate the family so that they believe that questions are unwelcome. Finally, information is power. It may be helpful to select one or two people to whom information will be conveyed, but situations must be avoided where one family member is controlling the flow of information to the remainder of the family.

Some families are risk adverse, whereas others tolerate a great deal of risk. It is helpful to discern what weight the family attaches to small probabilities. For example, if there is a "5% chance" of the patient leaving the intensive care unit or the hospital alive, some families will want every intervention so that chance can be realized, and others will conclude that the potential benefit is not worth the known burdens. Of course, in making decisions on behalf of a patient, it is helpful to know the patient's own risk characteristics. In these situations, it also should be noted that some physicians avoid risks and others take them, even where the chance of success is minute.

A family may hold onto an initial favorable prognosis despite further events, or may not recognize that medicine is an art and that sometimes exact diagnosis is not possible, or may not understand multiple diagnoses where some are more serious than others. Some families, especially some religious families, do not tolerate uncertainty well.[6] Consultants may disagree on substantive issues, or do not read each other's progress notes. Consider, for example, a situation in which dialysis is not physiologically futile and is recommended by one physician, but its provision should be considered in light of the patient's overall condition and prognosis. A family member also may latch on to one consultant's positive information to the exclusion of negative information provided by other consultants. This becomes most obvious when certain favorable medical terms or phrases are repeated like mantras, so that new information is simply not assimilated. A chaplain should be able to determine when this is happening.

A family who is resisting the withdrawal of life-sustaining interventions may simply need time to adjust to the patient's impending death, and to express their feelings of guilt, anger, sadness, frustration, and grief. It may take time and patience to understand a family's resistance, and a chaplain can be of assistance. Time trials are important, as is setting the day and time that interventions will be withdrawn in order to allow for family members to gather, to determine who will be present, and to give time for rituals such as sacramental anointing.[7]

It is essential to establish that any religious reason for resisting the withdrawal of life support be based on the patient's religious beliefs, not those of other family members. Religious reasons can mask other conscious or unconscious motives. Problematic situations arise, for example, when the patient was raised in a religious tradition, and the parents who are adherents to that tradition dispute the patient's present beliefs with the patient's spouse.[8] A chaplain can help to discern exactly what are the patient's beliefs and to facilitate the parents and spouse to come to a mutual understanding.

An intervention that would clearly be inappropriate based on personal preference or one of the reasons given above does not become appropriate just because it is backed by a sincerely held religious belief.[9] Established religious beliefs should receive more weight than personal preference, but, in exchange, they should be held to a higher evidentiary standard. Therefore, it is important to be able to distinguish between an idiosyncratic belief and a religious belief in order to make clinical decisions.[10] Many religious traditions have a specific doctrine or a body of theology concerning inappropriate medical interventions, and a chaplain can be very helpful in assisting the family to apply it to the situation at hand, as well as explaining it to the physician. However, some religious traditions are grounded in experience rather than in doctrine, and it is easy to discriminate against these traditions as irrational. The fact is that the ultimate ground of religious belief is faith in the supernatural, and is therefore unscientific. In short, it is unreasonable to require religious beliefs to be rational in the sense of being scientific, but it is reasonable to require them to be congruent with the religious tradition's established doctrine, or, for those traditions that do not have an established doctrine, with the relevant practice of the religious community. In other words, religious views should be tested and validated, and there should be verification that a belief is consistent with the patient's religious tradition. However sincerely a belief is held, it is not an adequate basis for resistance to the withdrawal of life-sustaining interventions if it is not internally coherent.

Many mainstream Christian churches teach that God uses suffering to bring the sufferer to repentance and salvation. Suffering is a mark of God's love, not of God's anger. This belief may help a patient who is responsive and can bring meaning to his suffering, but a patient cannot repent if he is unresponsive and further medical treatment is inappropriate. That suffering may be evidence of God's love or redemptive by nature does not necessarily mean that suffering should be tolerated or even extended.[11]

In addition, many people are confused about the doctrine of their professed religious tradition. For example, some Roman Catholics will resist withdrawal of life-sustaining interventions because they believe that the Catholic position on the beginning of life translates into a vitalist stand on the end of life. In fact, since 1957, the Catholic Church has permitted the withdrawal of life-sustaining interventions where the burden of the interventions is disproportionate to the benefit received.[12] There is also a discrepancy when a family member believes that her religious tradition forbids the withdrawal of life-sustaining interventions when it only gently discourages it.[13] In some cases, there is a difference between the explicit theology of the believer's tradition and the believer's implicit theology and private image of God, which may or may not be unconscious. For example, some family members may believe that God is harsh and judgmental and that suffering is God's retribution for the individual sin of the patient or for their sin; as a consequence, they may be reluctant to agree to the withdrawal of life-sustaining interventions in order to stave off God's judgment. This belief may particularly affect the family when the patient has intended suicide, and, unfortunately, there are occasions where a minister or priest supports this belief. A chaplain often can help family members to come to a greater understanding of the theology of their religious tradition.[14]

There are several religious beliefs that can conflict with the fact that medical treatment is inappropriate in certain situations. The first is the belief that only God can take a life, and doctors are not God. A chaplain may be able to discuss with the family the possibility that medical treatment is standing in the way of God's plan for the patient. Another conflicting belief is that the patient must be kept on life-sustaining interventions so that God has time to perform a miracle. The members of the medical team may not personally believe that divine action can transcend the laws of nature, but the patient's bedside is not the place to dispute the belief in miracles. A belief in the omnipotence of God implies a belief in miracles. However, the application of that general power is not always specific or particular, and because experience teaches to the contrary, there is no assurance in any given case that God will perform a miracle. A chaplain may be able to assist a family to discern when such a belief betrays a lack of confidence in God's power or a desire to manipulate God, for it is unreasonable to declare that an omnipotent God needs a ventilator or another day in order to perform a miracle.

Some religious traditions that are grounded in the experience of the Holy Spirit have a dualistic view of nature. God is good, but demonic spirits exist which are evil, and there is a constant battle between good and evil for souls as well as for physical health. The spirits of illness may prevent healing, and must be battled in prayer. Life-sustaining interventions cannot be withdrawn until the evil spirit has been vanquished and there has been a physical healing. To an outsider, sometimes family members seem to be more concerned about battling evil spirits than they are with the patient's suffering.[15] There is a related belief that health is a promise of God, and that a believer need only speak that promise in order to claim it; death is possible only when belief fails.[16] In these cases, a family may resist the withdrawal of life-sustaining interventions because death implies a failure of belief.

In conclusion, suffering is meaningless under either one of two conditions: the first condition is that the patient lacks the resources to make it meaningful, and the second is that medical interventions that either cause or enable the suffering are inappropriate. From a spiritual and religious perspective, meaningless suffering is an evil, and that fact has implications for life-sustaining interventions. The value of biological life always should be measured against the meaningfulness of the suffering that is necessary to sustain it. A physician cannot acquiesce to a family who resists the withdrawal of life-sustaining interventions where these interventions serve only to sustain biological life in the face of meaningless suffering. When the patient's suffering is reframed for the family in this way, and their resistance is met with patience and reason, most families will come to terms and act with kindness, if not with understanding.

References

1. I consider an intervention inappropriate when, quantitatively, it has a minute likelihood of success, that is, it probably will not postpone death for more than a few days,

or when, qualitatively, it is outside the standard of practice, although the two are not equivalent. *See*, Robert D. Orr and Leigh B. Genesen, "Requests for 'inappropriate' treatment based on religious beliefs." *Journal of Medical Ethics* 1997;23:142. The determination that the known risks of the burdens of an intervention outweigh the potential benefits is an ethical one, but such a determination would necessarily mean that the intervention in question is inappropriate.

2. From an ethical standpoint, there is no difference between withdrawing and withholding life-sustaining interventions. However, for some families, there is a greater psychological resistance to withdrawing as opposed to withholding interventions.

3. Ann Alpers and Bernard Lo, "Avoiding family feuds: responding to surrogate demands for life-sustaining interventions." 27 J.L. Med & Ethics 74 (Spring 1999). Instances of substituted judgment will be excluded, where the patient's views are known and faithfully reported to his physician. Note that it is an open question whether the substituted judgment standard differs substantially from the best interests standard in actual practice.

4. I believe that waking a patient so that the family can say goodbye is inappropriate because it violates the consent requirement and the principle of beneficence, *inter alia. See*, Anna Batchelor, Leslie Jenal, Farhad Kapadia, Stephen Streat, Leslie Whetsine, and Brian Woodcock, "Ethics roundtable debate: should a sedated dying patient be wakened to say goodbye to family?" *Critical Care* 2003, 7. This article is available online at http://ccforum.com/inpress/cc2329.

5. This is one reason why family presence at a resuscitation attempt can decrease anxiety and worry that "everything" has not been done.

6. Harold G. Koenig, Michael E. McCullough, and David B. Larson, *Handbook of religion and health*. Oxford: Oxford University Press; 2001:74.

7. Ideally, nurses who have developed a relationship with the family should be present, and monitors should be turned off.

8. This was the case with Terry Schiavo.

9. I strongly disagree with the contrary position taken by Robert D. Orr and Leigh B. Genesen in "Requests for 'inappropriate' treatment based on religious beliefs."

10. Alpers and Lo.

11. For a discussion of the redemptive nature of suffering, *see*, United States Conference of Catholic Bishops, *Ethical and religious directives for catholic health care services*. 4th ed. Washington, DC: National Conference of Catholic Bishops; 2001:§ 5. The directives are online at http://www.usccb.org/bishops/directives.shtml.

12. Pius XII, Address to an International Group of Physicians (February 24, 1957); Sacred Congregation for the Doctrine of the Faith, *Declaration On Euthanasia* (May 5, 1980), § IV; John Paul II, Encyclical Letter *Evangelium Vitae* (March 25, 1995), § 65 ("To forego extraordinary or disproportionate means is not the equivalent of suicide or euthanasia; it rather expresses acceptance of the human condition in the face of death").

13. James F Buryska, "Assessing the ethical weight of cultural, religious and spiritual claims in the clinical context." *Journal of Medical Ethics* 2001;27:118.

14. It is often helpful to use the New Testament for Christians. *See*, for example, Luke 13:1, John 9.

15. *See*, David M. Smolin, "Praying For Baby Rena: religious liberty, medical futility, and miracles." 25 Seton Hall L. Rev. 960 (1995).

16. Koenig, McCullough, and Larson, 55.

Pharmacotherapy Considerations during End-of-Life Care of Critically Ill Adults

Amy Roach and Ted L. Rice

> To cure sometimes, to relieve often, to comfort always.
>
> —Hippocrates of Cos (circa 400 B.C.E.)
>
> We must all die. But that I can save him from days of torture, that is what I feel as my great and ever new privilege.
>
> —Albert Schweitzer (1875–1965)

It is simply unacceptable for critically ill patients to suffer while undergoing end-of-life care (EOLC) in the intensive-care unit (ICU), and the prevention or alleviation of any pain, anxiety, or dysphoria is of paramount importance to the patient, his loved ones, and the entire healthcare team.[1–3] Our society places a very high value on self-determination, and when a patient or their surrogate chooses to discontinue or forego life-sustaining treatments or procedures, healthcare providers must modify their care plan from a curative strategy to one that assures that the patient will die with dignity and in comfort. In a study of 206 mechanically ventilated ICU patients who received morphine, midazolam, and lorazepam during withdrawal of life support, 91% of family members interviewed believed that the patient was either totally, very, or mostly comfortable.[4] Indeed, it has been proposed that failure to plan for and provide compassionate EOLC is tantamount to medical malpractice.[5] Although there are a number of comforting strategies available, such as music, guided imagery, and psychotherapy, we will only address the relative merits of pharmacotherapeutic agents used in the management of adult EOLC patients. Because of space limitations, we will not discuss EOLC for critically ill pediatric patients, other than to note that physicians in The Netherlands not only withhold life-sustaining therapies in severely ill newborn infants but also actively hasten death.[6]

Applying the basic principles of pain management to assist in meeting EOLC patient-centered goals can be accomplished effectively when the healthcare provider has a sound knowledge of pharmacology and pharmacokinetics. There are a number of tools that can be used to assess the degree of pain, sedation, and agitation in patients, such as visual analog scales, the Riker Sedation-Agitation Scale (SAS), the Motor Activity Assessment Scale (MAAS), the Ramsay Scale, and the Confusion Assessment Method for the Intensive Care Unit (CAM-ICU).[7,8] The assessment of pain and suffering in EOLC patients who are not awake and alert is challenging and often relies on evaluating physiologic signs of distress, such as tachypnea or gasping, hypertension, diaphoresis, and agitation. Healthcare practitioners use these signs to assess the patient's degree of pain and suffering, often in cooperation with the patient's family. Based on these assessments, the healthcare practitioner can select or modify pharmacotherapeutic strategies during EOLC.

The types of agents used most commonly in EOLC include parenteral analgesics, sedative-hypnotics, neuroleptics, antiemetics, and anticholinergics. This is in contrast to palliative care of the hospice patient where oral agents are the preferred routes of administration. The pharmacotherapy regimen must be designed to provide adequate comfort, even if dose escalation might hasten death as an unintended consequence. Although there are data that indicate that this principle of double effect, where analgesics are used to relieve pain and hasten death, may not occur.[9,10] In addition, opioids are remarkably safe, and patients can tolerate unusually large doses, as in a patient who required 1650 mg of morphine per hour.[11] It should be noted that the use of neuromuscular blocking agents, such as pancuronium, cisatracurium, or succinylcholine, during EOLC is contraindicated. They have no analgesic or sedative properties and may prevent recognition of the physiologic signs of pain or suffering.

Analgesics[7,12]

Opioids have long been the mainstay to treat pain and suffering. Opiates are μ-receptor agonists that produce analgesia, sedation, respiratory depression, constipation, urinary retention, nausea, and euphoria. The Society of Critical Care Medicine has identified morphine as the preferred opioid analgesic agent for use in the ICU, with hydromorphone and fentanyl as alternatives. Morphine is the most frequently used opioid analgesic in the United States because of its low cost, potency, and analgesic efficacy. Following intravenous (IV) administration, morphine has a half-life of 1.5 to 2 hours and reaches its peak effect within 5 minutes. Allergic reaction is commonly related to histamine release, especially when it is administered rapidly. In contrast, fentanyl is a synthetic opioid with 80 to 100 times the potency of morphine. It results in less sedation, less histamine release, and less hypotension. Unlike morphine, fentanyl has a half-life of 30 to 60 minutes because of rapid distribution. It too reaches its peak effect within 5 minutes of administration, making frequent dosing possible, a common theme following terminal wean and extubation. Meperidine should not be used for sedation or pain management during EOLC because of the potential for neurotoxicity from its metabolite, normeperidine.

Sedative-Hypnotics[7,12]

Benzodiazepines have long been indicated for induction of general anesthesia, continuous sedation in intubated and ventilated patients, just prior to invasive procedures, and for the treatment of status epilepticus. The desirable effects produced by members of this drug class for EOLC include amnesia and anxiolysis. Benzodiazepines work synergistically with opioids and can be very helpful in the prevention of premorbid seizures. Midazolam is a short-acting benzodiazepine that rapidly penetrates the central nervous system to exert its effects quickly, much like diazepam. Unfortunately, the drug has a very brief duration of action and must be used as a continuous infusion to maintain adequate sedation when used for EOLC. Lorazepam is an intermediate-acting benzodiazepine and is more attractive for use in EOLC in the ICU. Its peak effect is approximately 30 minutes after IV administration and is not altered by hepatic or renal dysfunction. In contrast to midazolam, lorazepam can be administered by intermittent IV bolus rather than by continuous IV infusion.

Propofol is a very attractive sedative for use in the mechanically ventilated patient and as an anesthetic largely due to its very short pharmacodynamic effects. Following IV bolus administration, the sedative effect terminates because of rapid distribution out of the central nervous system. When propofol is administered by continuous IV infusion, it can be titrated to achieve varying levels of sedation and unconsciousness. Hypotension is the major adverse effect associated with propofol administration, it has IV incompatibility problems, and because it can support microbial growth there is a potential for contamination and subsequent patient infection. Propofol has no analgesic effects, similar to barbiturates, which have been associated with euthanasia when given at EOLC.

Dexmedetomidine is a selective α-2-receptor agonist that is FDA approved for postoperative sedation for up to 24 hours, but has been used for sedation in ICU patients for longer periods.[13] It provides analgesic, sedative, and anxiolytic effects without significant respiratory depression. An important advantage for dexmedetomidine is that it allows the patient to be maintained in a twilight state and to be easily awakened. Its use in EOLC has yet to be clearly identified.

Neuroleptics[7,12]

Delirium is defined as an acute confusional state that can be difficult to differentiate from anxiety. Patients can experience delirium during EOLC. The administration of opioids or benzodiazepines can worsen the symptoms of delirium, and it is important to differentiate delirium from anxiety. Pharmacologic management of delirium at end of life should be gauged toward patient comfort rather than toward complete resolution of the delirium.

Haloperidol has proven efficacy in the treatment of delirium. Dosing can be increased every 30 minutes until relief of patient's symptoms because it does not possess significant sedative effects. The primary disadvantage in using haloperidol is the risk of extrapyramidal symptoms; however the length of drug therapy in EOLC is often quite short thus decreasing this risk.

Anticholinergics and Antiemetics

Anticholinergics play an important role in symptom management during EOLC. As respiratory failure ensues following terminal wean and extubation, gurgling or wet-sounding breathing is a common finding. Saliva often collects in the back of patient's throats and they are unable to swallow it or effectively expectorate it. This saliva collection can produce an unpleasant sound during breathing, often referred to as the death rattle, and can be one of the most uncomfortable and disturbing signs for family members. The antisecretory effects of anticholinergic drugs can be useful to depress salivary and bronchial secretions while dilating the bronchi. Common anticholinergics used during EOLC include glycopyrolate, hyoscyamine sulfate, and scopolamine.

Nausea and vomiting have been frequently reported in patients during EOLC. Leaving nasogastric tubes in place or placing one intentionally to relieve nausea and vomiting results in patient discomfort. The use of antiemetic agents is a better option for symptom management. Choosing the most appropriate for use during EOLC requires some thought by the healthcare team. Drugs such as metoclopramide, prochlorperazine, and promethazine are excellent choices because of their antiemetic effects, sedation enhancement, and central nervous system depression. These antiemetics act synergistically with narcotics and sedatives. Metoclopramide helps to accelerate gastric emptying, thus resulting in less nausea and decreases the chance of emesis, however, it also increases intestinal transit of secretions and may produce diarrhea. Promethazine is a histamine H-1 receptor blocker and decreases the adverse effects associated with histamine release, such as increased mucous production, coryza, and conjunctivitis. Ondansetron has long been known to be very effective in treating nausea and vomiting associated with administration of antineoplastic chemotherapy. It has an immediate onset of action; however, it does not possess sedative or anticholinergic properties.

Summary

Healthcare providers in ICU settings are committed to providing diagnostic and therapeutic procedures for critically ill patients that are intended to cure or mitigate disease or trauma. When the patient's condition becomes irreversible and additional treatment would be medically futile, implementation of EOLC with an emphasis on pain relief and comforting measures is indicated. Pharmacotherapeutic agents provide the most reliable and effective method to attain EOLC goals. We have provided the dosing strategies recommended from the UPMC Presbyterian-Shadyside Comfort Measures Only order form.

References

1. Steinhauser KE, Christakis NA, Clipp EC, et al. Factors considered important at the end of life by patients, family, physicians, and other care providers. JAMA 2000;284:2476–2482.
2. Clarke EB, Luce JM, Curtis JR, et al. A content analysis of forms, guidelines, and other materials documenting end-of-life care in intensive care units. J Crit Care 2004;19:108–117.
3. Heyland DK, Rocker GM, O'Callaghan CJ, et al. Dying in the ICU: perspectives of family members. Chest 2003;124:392–397.
4. Rocker GM, Heyland DK, Cook DJ, et al. Most critically ill patients are perceived to die in comfort during withdrawal of life support: a Canadian multicentre study. Can J Anesth 2004;51:623–630.
5. Lynn J. Goldstein NE. Advance care planning for fatal chronic illness: avoiding commonplace errors and unwarranted suffering. Ann Intern Med 2003;138:812–818.
6. Verhagen E, Sauer PJJ. The Groningen protocol — euthanasia in severely ill newborns. N Engl J Med 2005;352:959–962.
7. Jacobi J, Fraser GL, Coursin DB, et al. Clinical practice guidelines for the sustained use of sedatives and analgesics in the critically ill adult. Crit Care Med 2002;30:119–141.
8. Ely EW, Margolin R, Francis J, et al. Evaluation of delirium in critically ill patients: validation of the Confusion Assessment Method for the Intensive Care Unit (CAM-ICU). Crit Care Med 2001;29:1370–1379.
9. Thoms A, Sykes N. Opioid use in last week of life and implications for end-of-life decision making. Lancet 2000;356:398–399.
10. Chan JD, Treece PD, Engelberg RA, et al. Narcotic and benzodiazepine use after withdrawal of life support. Association with time to death? Chest 2004;126:286–293.
11. Donahue SR. Morphine sulfate intravenous dose of 1650 mg per hour. Hosp Pharm 1989;24:311.
12. Truog RD, Cist AF, Brackett SE, et al. Recommendations for end-of-life care in the intensive care unit: The Ethics Committee of the Society of Critical Care Medicine. Crit Care Med 2001;29:2332–2348.
13. Shehabi Y, Ruettimann U, Adamson H, et al. Dexmedetomidine infusion for more than 24 hours in critically ill patients: sedative and cardiovascular effects. Intensive Care Med 2004; 30(12):2188–2196.

13
The Intensive Care Unit of the Future

Mike Darwin and Brian Wowk

> It is the business of the future to be dangerous.... The major advances in civilization are processes that all but wreck the societies in which they occur.
>
> —Alfred North Whitehead
>
> The only way to predict the future is to have power to shape the future.
>
> —Eric Hoffer

Introduction

The *ultimate* future of critical care medicine is surprisingly easy to predict with certainty. The difference between a healthy person and ill one can be reduced to the difference in the way their atoms are arranged. From a broken bone to a broken strand of DNA, illness is ultimately reducible to how the structures that embody life are configured and interact with each other. Today's clinicians can only affect events going on in their patients at the molecular level mostly in indirect ways. We have a little specificity, but no precision. We can introduce molecules (drugs) that turn or on or off certain genes, activate certain molecular mechanisms, or derange or shut down others. Antibiotics do this to flora we consider undesirable or out of control in the patient. Steroids and many other drugs signal genes or, like the pressors, more immediately act on cell machinery. We can poison metabolism and disrupt DNA with chemotherapy and radiation, but we lack the ability, at least clinically, to reset the DNA of a neoplastic cell to its healthy state.

On the macroscopic level we can pinch hit for ventilation, renal function, and even circulation, but our ability to repair or replace severely damaged organs is limited to acquiring them from a naturally "engineered" source via transplantation. No laws of physics speak against nanoscale engineering and, in the fullness of time, it is inevitable (providing we and our technological progress both survive) that we will someday build cell and tissue repair devices that act at the molecular level. The nature and capabilities of such nanoscale medicine are already broadly understood. Indeed, we are today in much the same position Leonardo da Vinci was in 500 years ago.[1] Da Vinci was able to envision most mechanical devices we know of today, but was unable to build them. He designed countless machines with ball bearings — but the hardened steel needed to fabricate durable, pressure-resistant ball bearings was 300 years in the future.

The Day after Tomorrow: Nanomedicine?

In the mid-1980s, the scanning tunneling microscope (STM) was developed,[2] allowing us for the first time to "see" atoms, and much more importantly, to manipulate them with precision. As the 1989 picture in Figure 13-1 illustrates, it became possible for the first time in human history to manipulate atoms with precision. Since that time it has been possible to design, but not yet build, molecular bearings (Fig. 13-2) as well as countless other nanoscale devices (Fig. 13-3).[3]

The logical endpoint of molecular nanotechnology is the construction of cell and tissue repair devices capable of manipulating the atoms comprising living matter with atomic precision. This is the ultimate future of critical care medicine and the end of aging and disease as we currently understand it.

Long before devices such as the one shown in Figure 13-4 are ever fabricated, medicine will have simpler tools acquired by modifying natural structures. As an example, researchers at the Scripps Institute have reengineered the Cowpea mosaic virus (CPMV; a plant virus) by integrating internalin B (a surface protein on bacteria that facilitates entry of the microorganisms into mammalian

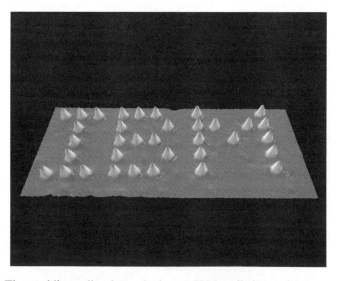

FIG. 13-1. The world's smallest logo; the letters IBM spelled out with 35 xenon atoms on a nickel crystal. (Reprinted courtesy of International Business Machines Corporation, copyright 1990 © International Business Machines Corporation.)

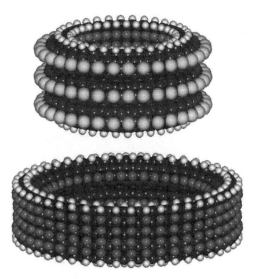

FIG. 13-2. Molecular bearing (disassembled). (Image courtesy of Ralph C. Merkle.)

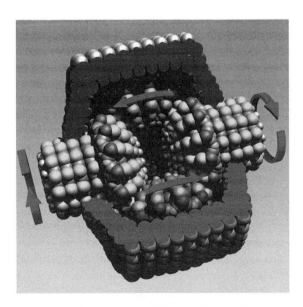

FIG. 13-3. A cutaway view of a molecular differential gear. All components are strong covalent solids modeled using molecular mechanics methods. The shafts are constrained to turn in opposite directions relative to the casing by the meshing of surface ridges on six gears. (Design by K. Eric Drexler with R. Merkle. Image prepared using NanoEngineer and POVray.)

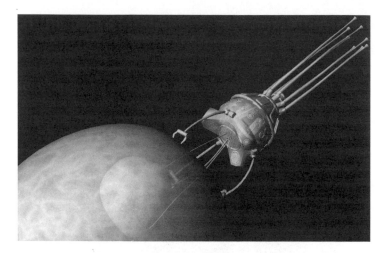

FIG. 13-4. Artist's conception of a cell repair device. (Image by Yuriy Svidinenko of Nanotechnology News Network.)

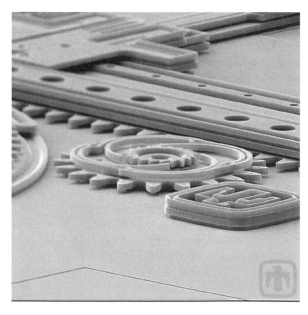

FIG. 13-5. Ultramicroscopic rack and pinion; the gear teeth are 6 microns in diameter, a little smaller than a red blood cell. This device exists as a working prototype today. (Image by Sandia National Laboratories.)

cells) and herstatin (a cancer inhibitor that recognizes HER2, a cancer-related cell-surface receptor) into the viral capsid. This allows the virus to bind to mammalian cells and introduce drug molecules or other "cargo" into cells.

The investigators have even selectively removed the viral RNA from the viral capsid, creating a hollow interior which allows for loading of even more cargo.[4,5] They were also able to create a port in the capsid which can be opened or closed to allow for loading and unloading cargo to be delivered to selectively targeted cells.

So, while it possible to broadly predict with confidence what the distant future of critical care medicine will be, it is not possible to predict when it will come to pass (Fig. 13-5).

But What of the Day after Today?

By far the most difficult task is not to look into the far future, but to anticipate what will (or should) follow from where we are today. Where will critical medicine be in the next decade or the decade after that? To see into that future we must try and distinguish between what is possible and what will, in fact, happen. There is a vast difference between that which is technologically possible from that which is socially and politically desirable, or even acceptable. We are now 6 years into the 21st century and it is only necessary to screen Arthur C. Clarke's and Stanley Kubrick's film *2001: A Space Odyssey*, to understand the dichotomy between technological possibility and sociopolitical priorities. Clarke's technological vision of the world in 2001 is completely valid, in that it envisioned technology which violates no physical law, and which relies on the reasoned application of insights and understanding already at hand. Clarke was "right" about the future of the communications satellite (his invention first described in a letter to the editor in February 1945 issue of *Wireless World*[6]) and wrong about a von Braun–style space station, a lunar base, and a manned expedition to the moons of Jupiter. The "problem" was not with the technology, but with the desires and priorities of the civilization that wielded it.

In attempting to predict the near future of critical care medicine it would be a fool's errand to try and do better than Arthur C. Clarke did in envisioning the future of the human exploration and colonization of space.

Defining the Discipline

Critical care medicine attempts to salvage individuals injured beyond all possibility of natural, nontechnologically assisted repair and healing. The hallmark of the intensive care unit (ICU) patient is injury or illness so profound that he has lost the ability to maintain homeostasis or sustain other vital functions such as gas exchange, circulation, digestion, host defense, and excretion of waste products. The ICU is thus a place where currently immature and costly technologies, such as mechanical ventilation, extracorporeal membrane oxygenation (ECMO), application of pressors, intra-aortic balloon pumps (IABPs), left ventricular assist devices (LVADs), tube-facilitated enteral nutrition, total parenteral nutrition (TPN), antimicrobial therapy, and renal replacement therapy (RRT), are in play.

The physician–philosopher Lewis Thomas described three levels of technology in the evolution of medicine: nontechnology (palliation and caring), halfway technology (fails to address the root cause of the pathology), and high technology (definitively addresses the cause of the pathology at a molecular level and prevents or reverses it, as described in the opening of this article). Thomas describes halfway technology as "... a level of technology (that) is, by its nature, at the same time highly sophisticated and profoundly primitive. It is the kind of thing that one must continue to do until there is a genuine understanding of the mechanisms involved in disease."[7] This description almost perfectly defines the practice of contemporary critical care medicine.

The High Cost of Halfway Technology

As of the year 2000, critical care medicine consumed 4.2% of US healthcare costs and 0.56% of the US gross domestic product.[8] While there are data that indicate the cost effectiveness of critical care medicine is comparable to that achieved in other areas of medicine,[9] there is no doubt that critical care medicine is a bad bargain and an extravagance when compared to the value returned for dollars invested in basic public health infrastructure. The Cambridge dictionary defines a luxury as "something expensive which is pleasant to have but is not necessary," and it is worth noting that an antonym for luxury is *necessity*. Critical care medicine is unarguably a necessity for those individuals in need of it. However, most patients who utilize critical care medicine in the West do not pay for it on fee-for-service basis. Rather, government administered healthcare programs or large bureaucratic insurance companies pay the tab and determine what kinds of technology are worthwhile. Thus, access to, and expansion of, critical care medicine is subject to its cost–benefit ratio to society at large. As the population of the developed world ages, the demand for halfway technologies is exploding. The effect of public health, preventive medicine (including dietary changes, statins, and aggressive screening for and treatment of hypertension and diabetes), and more effective treatment of early onset degenerative diseases has resulted in a profound extension of mean lifespan. Mean lifespan in the West has doubled since 1900[10] and may well approach the maximum human lifespan of 100 to 120 years in the next three decades.[11]

Extension of the mean lifespan, absent extension of the maximum lifespan, is also of necessity a halfway technology, because this approach fails to effect the fundamental reason for loss of vitality and ultimately death: the pathology of senescence. Many gerontologists and other physicians argue that aging is not a disease and seek to "square the curve" by allowing people to remain healthy until almost the day they reach the maximum human lifespan.[12] Once this "natural" milestone is reached the patient is supposed to more or less instantly disintegrate, like Oliver Wendell Holmes' *Wonderful One Hoss Shay*:[13] "That was built in such a logical way... it went to pieces all at once, — All at once, and nothing first, — Just as bubbles do when they burst... You see, of course, if you're not a dunce. End of the wonderful one-hoss shay. — Logic is logic. That's all I say."

But as Holmes well knew, aging is not a process wherein organs and tissues function perfectly until they disintegrate "As if (they) had been to the mill and ground!" In this case the dunces are those physicians and scientists who fail to realize the obvious; that aging is a steady loss of essential reserve capacity with many parts of the organism experiencing undesirable and costly failures prior to failure of the system as a whole and that compression of morbidity into the last few months or even year or two of life is not likely. As long as the fundamental mechanisms that underlie the aging process remain beyond our control the demand for increasingly sophisticated and costly halfway medicine will continue to grow. This is the perspective from which I will attempt to predict technological future of critical care medicine.

The Pace of Technological Advance

As Kurzweil has elegantly pointed out, the pace of *most* technological advance is at least exponential even across paradigm shifts such as the evolution of information handling technology from telegraphy in circa 1900 through the integrated circuit today (Fig. 13-6).[14]

The generation and penetration of a broad range of new technologies has also been surprisingly smoothly exponential, as Kurzweil shows in the graph in Figure 13-7.

Nor is this rate of progress confined to computer science or information handling technologies; it holds true for the biological sciences as is reflected in the exponential growth and reduction of cost in sequencing the human genome (Fig. 13-8).

Extrapolating progress at the *current* exponential rate, Kurzweil notes that the next 100 years of human progress will equate to 20,000 years of progress! However, there is selectivity in the examples Kurzweil chooses which may have profound implications for attempts to predict the future of critical care medicine.

Origins and Costs of Overregulation

Both medicine and government-operated space programs share two common features: an overwhelming need for innovative technology and a nearly complete intolerance for its catastrophic failure. Frequent and often catastrophic

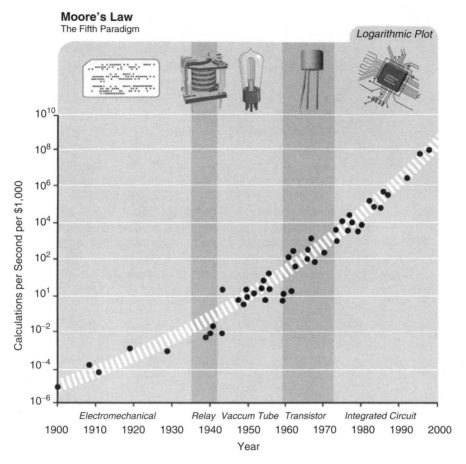

FIG. 13-6. Moore's law demonstrates the exponential increase in the growth of computing capability over a period of a century. (Image courtesy of Ray Kurzweil, author of the Singularity is Near.)

failures are the handmaiden of rapid technological advance. Rapid advances due to intense experimentation at the cost of many false starts and failures characterized the history of aviation, computer science, consumer electronics, and early critical care medicine. Areas of endeavor where risk is eschewed, and failure considered unacceptable, typically become subject to heavy government regulation. Such regulation slows, stops, or even reverses technological progress.

Pharmaceutical innovation under the aegis of the US Food and Drug Administration (FDA) has long been drastically inhibited due to byzantine paperwork and astronomical costs. FDA regulation has been getting progressively more complex and costly, so much so that today it takes 12 to 15 years to develop a drug and navigate the approval process — with no guarantee of approval. The average cost of introducing a new drug into the market place is

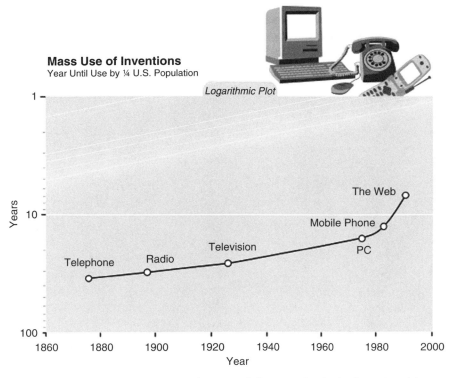

FIG. 13-7. The increase in the penetration rate of diverse technologies from electricity to the Internet also follows a fairly exponential curve. (Image courtesy of Ray Kurzweil, author of the Singularity is Near.)

now approaching half a billion dollars. These astronomical numbers become understandable when the breakdown of this cost is considered. Currently, an average of 60 clinical trials is required for each new drug before it is even eligible for FDA approval and marketing.[15]

This does not include the very considerable burden of conducting ongoing clinical trials to maintain licensing for existing, approved drugs or to expand their use in conditions for which they were not originally approved. To put this into perspective, 85% of the cost of pharmaceutical development is expended complying the FDA regulations dealing with safety and efficacy. This does not include the very substantial burden imposed by Good Manufacturing Practice (GMP) regulations, which apply to every aspect of the manufacturing process from how raw materials are stored, tracked, processed, and so on, through to the arrival of the completed device or drug at its point of use.

Nor does this take into consideration the blizzard of costly and time-consuming paperwork associated with adverse event reporting: a system which requires a lengthy report on every misuse, malfunction, adverse reaction, or unexpected outcome in every device or medication a company has manufactured and distributed. A blood pump or heart–lung resuscitator sold in 1976,

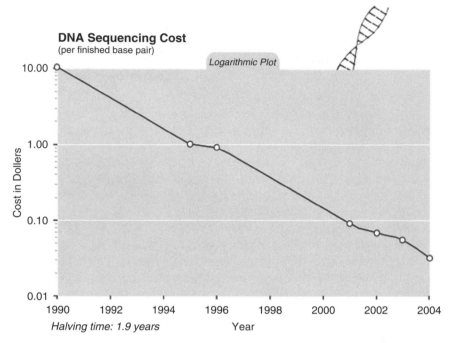

FIG. 13-8. Nonclinical biomedical technology such as DNA sequencing, being largely unregulated, also advances exponentially. (Image courtesy of Ray Kurzweil, author of the Singularity is Near.)

and never maintained since the day it was put into service, is subject to the same adverse event reporting as a newly manufactured product the company sold today. If the FDA was really protecting the consumer from widespread and costly disasters, the value of the benefit of regulation might be worth it. However, the reverse seems to the case. As the Cato Institute 2005 Report to Congress notes:

> The effect of FDA regulation on the price of drugs is profound. Assuming a 14 percent return on drug development, excessive FDA regulation increases the required break-even return on a drug by about 200 percent. Not only do such regulatory costs raise the price of new drugs, they also reduce basic research at a time when the opportunities for medical progress are increasing.[16]

Impact of Regulation on the Progress of Medicine

The impact of choking regulation on medical progress can perhaps best be illustrated by what happened to the medical device industry. In 1976, the FDA began aggressively regulating medical devices of all kinds: tongue depressors (class I), software and imaging technology (class II), and pacemakers and ventilators (class III). Even the development of telemedicine was virtually stopped in its tracks when the FDA ruled that all components of the system, including the transmission devices (land lines, satellites, software, cameras, sound and packet data transmission) were medical devices and subject to the same costly regulatory constraints as are products like artificial hearts and implantable defibrillators. Rapidly evolving innovation in this area was brought to a virtual standstill.

The period from ~1940 to 1976 marked a veritable explosion of critical care medicine technologies, particularly in the arena of devices which were minimally regulated at that time. It is worth considering these technologies and reflecting on the nature of subsequent developments.

- Endotracheal intubation became widespread after the use of curare became routine in the early 1940s.[17] Succinylcholine was first synthesized in 1949 and was in wide use by the mid-1950s.[18]
- A plethora of mechanical ventilators flooded the market, providing a wide range of choices. The natural weeding of the marketplace rapidly selected those devices that were affordable and effective and some, such as Bird series of ventilators, continue in use today.
- Cardiac catheterization was first demonstrated by Werner Forssmann in 1929 by the bold move of performing the procedure on himself with little or no assistance at a time when introducing artificial appliances into the beating heart was deemed likely, if not certain, to cause immediate cardiac fibrillation and death.[19] The procedure entered the realm of clinical medicine in 1941 with the work of Cournand and Richards, and, in 1956, Forssmann, Cournand, and Richards were awarded to Nobel Prize for its discovery.
- C. Walton Lillehei developed the first practical heart–lung machine using polyvinyl chloride (PVC) tubing used in the beer brewing industry in combination with a silicone antifoam agent used in food processing (Dow-Corning Antifoam A), which coated food-grade stainless steel pot scourers that converted foamed blood back into bubble-free oxygenated and carbon dioxide (CO_2) cleansed blood which could be pumped into the patient's arterial circulation.[20]
- Blaylock, Taussig and Thomas, Dewall, Lillehei, DeBakey, Dennis, Cooley, and Kay and Cross invented and manufactured an almost endless stream of critical medical devices. The first aortic root cannula were custom made in the hospital machine shop from stainless steel. The first venous cannula consisted of a machined, fenestrated, cone-shaped stainless steel tip, which was inserted into an appropriate length of food-grade PVC tubing or, more often, latex rubber "medical grade" tubing manufactured for use in surgical drains and bladder catheters.
- Chronic hemodialysis became a reality circa 1960 due to the combined efforts Kolff, Alwall, Scribner, and others.[21] In 1972, the End Stage Renal Disease (ESRD) program was implemented providing universal access to hemodialysis in the United States. In 2002 there were 309,000 patients on hemodialysis at a cost of of $25.24 billion dollars.[22] The number of hemodialysis patients is projected to double to 650,000 by 2010.

The Coming Explosion of Physiological Data Acquisition

These rapid and enormous technological strides were facilitated by unfettered and unregulated application of innovation to medicine. In areas of endeavor where the cost of failure is deemed acceptable, advance is both rapid and sustained. Nowhere is this more evident than in the areas of computing, software development, industrial data acquisition and process control, and consumer electronics. These areas consistently attract the best and brightest minds because of the lack of regulation, rapid transit of technology from idea stage to developed product, and the prospect of large financial reward for success.

Technological advances in areas unrelated to critical care medicine will increasingly allow for monitoring and control of diverse physiological parameters. Continuous monitoring of blood and parenchymal gases, pH, electrolytes, lactate, and other metabolites, as well virtually all aspects of respiratory function, are either currently in clinical use or soon will be. Real-time sensor arrays capable of continuous monitoring of circulating hormone and cytokine levels already exist in the laboratory and will likely become clinically available in the next decade.[23]

Continuous monitoring of a wide range of other physiological parameters has long been routine: core temperature, mean arterial pressure (MAP), central venous pressure (CVP), cardiac output (CO), systemic vascular resistance (SVR), central venous oxygen saturation (SVO_2), intracranial pressure (ICP), cerebral cortical perfusion, and intra-abdominal pressure via a transducer placed in the urinary bladder. Continuous measurement of gastric tonometery and pH are both approved technologies, although little used at this time. The immediately foreseeable future presents the possibility of continuous monitoring of vascular and tissue drug levels or of any molecule, native or synthetic, which is of clinical interest.

Continuous passive imaging of the lungs using the sound of air during inhalation and exhalation allows dynamic visualization of the lungs and diagnosis of pneumonia, space occupying lesions, pleural effusions, congestive heart failure, empyema, and pneumothorax. The question becomes, "What to do with all this data?" As was noted earlier, contemporary critical care medicine consists almost exclusively of artificially imposing homeostasis on the severely injured patient. ICUs are basically artificial homeostats where gas exchange, pH, mass exchange (nutrition and waste disposal), level of consciousness (LOC), and just about everything else need to be provided, to varying degrees, artificially, until the patient's intrinsic healing capability can make repairs and resume these functions. It is ludicrous to expect these to be managed by mere mortals on a minute-by-minute basis — indeed, it is *impossible*.

As the quality, quantity, and continuity of data have improved it is becoming apparent that replicating the body's tight control of homeostasis is critical to improving survival. Meticulous management of pH, blood glucose and electrolytes, nutrition, ventilation, and perfusion are all proving essential to decreased morbidity and mortality.

The quantity of data now available to clinician and the need to integrate, understand, interpret, and act on it in real time are beyond the capacity of human beings. People are too valuable, too slow, and at the same time not "smart" enough or vigilant enough to make the increasingly complex decisions required to rescue patients with serious and prolonged derangements in homeostasis.

Automakers, computer chip fabricators, and interplanetary spacecraft designers realized this a long time ago. No one expects the driver of an automobile to control the second-to-second changes in humidity, temperature, barometric pressure, air/fuel filter loading, acceleration, and the like, in order to optimize engine performance and maximize mileage. Similarly, an interplanetary spacecraft is so complicated, with so many processes and instruments operating independently, and yet networked and interdependent, that no human could possibly control them "manually" (Fig. 13-9). Complex spacecraft are also so distant that humans cannot control them from earth.

The increasing load of physiological data will simply swamp staff or compromise adequate control of other, equally important parameters. Any attempt to bring tighter control or focus on one parameter will compromise control of other equally or more important ones! Administration of therapeutic drugs (and ever changing indications for their use), fluid balance, gases

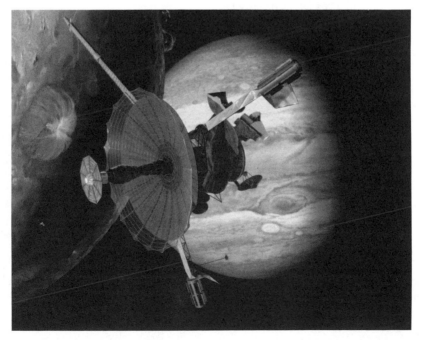

FIG. 13-9. The Galileo spacecraft autonomously manages vast quantities of data and controls dozens of complex internal systems (as well as its own navigation) using process control and primitive artificial intelligence technology

and pH, metabolic status, nutrition, management of ventilation, ICP, cerebral and systemic perfusion, intra-abdominal/intrathoracic pressure, management of renal replacement, drug interactions, optimum drug choices, *all* need to be brought under automated control under physician supervision.

Algorithms to manage these parameters based on data collected in real time need to replace short-term orders and the artificial intelligence (AI) system needs to be able to contact the treating physician(s) directly and ask for clarification or revision of orders (algorithms) if the patient is not responding as predicted or desired. All intravenous (IV)/enteral pumps, vents, RRT, pressors, *must* ultimately be managed on a minute-by-minute basis by intelligent, automated systems. This is now routine in automobiles, aircraft, complex integrated circuit chip production, and any other enormously complicated industrial procedure(s) involving feedback loops that must be addressed in real time, or something approaching it. The physician to his tastes and prejudices can tailor the content of the algorithms, however, the data will ultimately either validate or repudiate any given approach. *And* the data *will* be there.

This process should already be well underway in critical care medicine with the equivalent of gaming, process control, and consumer electronics programmers slaving away to design integrating platforms for all these modalities of data acquisition and control, in concert with the very best intensivists and researchers to generate algorithms for patient care in the ICU. Alas, this has not happened, not here in the West.

Zhongshan Hospital, Shanghai, China, 21 August 2025

Intensivist Dr. Shen Shuang had been notified the patient was en route from the operating room and had made the decision which ICU bay the patient would occupy only moments before he arrived. Aschwin van der Groot was a 39-year-old Dutch tourist who had suffered massive polytrauma in a motorcycle accident. En route to Zhongshan Hospital, he had hemorrhaged uncontrollably in the ambulance. By the time he reached the emergency department (ED) he was in cardiac arrest with a core temperature of 26°C. Over 11 liters of White Crane Oxyfluor perfluorocarbon emulsion blood substitute, chilled to 2°C, had been administered en route and then, as a last resort, 2 L of Ametabosol, a combination of cellular edema inhibiting polymers (polyglycerol and polyethylene glycol) and sugars [43] critical metabolites (phosphoenoyl pyruvate, diacyl glycerol) rTPA, a variety of potent free radical savengers (TEMPOL, PBN, melatonin) and, most critically, the small protein molecule known as Hibernation Induction Trigger (HIT). In the operating room (OR) he had been further cooled to 15°C using femoral–femoral cardiopulmonary bypass (CPB), buying additional time for the many surgical repairs needed. The patient required both a laparotomy and thoracotomy. Visceral injuries repaired were hollow viscus injuries of the ileum and bladder, splenectomy, stellate fracture of the liver, and right mainstem tracheobronchial disruption.

Open fractures of the right tibia and left humerus were reduced, and externally stabilized, and 11 lacerations were debrided and closed.

Following these repairs the patient was reperfused with whole blood to a hematocrit of 21% with a fluorocrit of 19%, rewarmed to 34°C, defibrillated, and acutely hemodynamically stabilized, at which time all surgical wounds were closed. Prior to transfer to the ICU, the patient was imaged (multimodal whole body scan with AI evaluation) in consultation with the hospital radiologist. The patient was not noted to have any previously unsuspected injuries and it was noted that central nervous system (CNS) perfusion was excellent. This was confirmed by the electrocortical monitoring array consisting of 30 small adhesive radio-friquency identification (RFID) sensors which, in addition to monitoring electroencephalographic parameters (EEG), also monitor Sp_{O2}, transcutaneous p_{O2}, pressure on the skin, and temperature. These RFID devices were powered by external radiofrequency energy that bathes the senors in energy providing both current for measurement and for transmission of the data back to the receiver.

The chronic care instrumentation and transport staff from the ICU was present in the OR suite as the patient's scans were completed. Their task was to instrument the patient for long-term care, transfer him to the integrated ICU care module (ICUCM) and transport him to the ICU. They began this procedure by applying additional RFID sensors over the ventral, dorsal, and lateral surfaces of the patient's body. Each adhesive sensor was peeled off its backing and attached to a predetermined area of the patient's body. The sensors were less than a millimeter thick, and looked like clear adhesive labels except for the exotic pattern of micron-scale circuitry and sensors surrounded by the RFID antennae.

These sensors would report pressure on the skin, local skin temperature, Sp_{O2}, and transcutaneous p_{O2}. Data from these sensors would be continuously transmitted to the ICUCM which uses this data to dynamically adjust the surface the patient rests on to prevent localized ischemia which might have resulted in pressure sores in the past.

The ICU transport team disconnects the patient's bladder catheter and connects it to the line in the ICUMC. The catheter does much more than drain urine. It is also a complex sensor array that continuously measures intra-abdominal pressure, temperature, and a wide range of metabolites and other compounds in the patient's urine. The catheter–sensor continuously checks for blood, bilirubin, dozens of both physiological and drug metabolites as well as total urine production, concentration, pH, and other variables which not only provide a continuous picture of renal function, but also of a wide array of biochemical and metabolic processes going on throughout the patient's body.

RFID sensors placed on the patient's chest also acquire EKG data from over 40 leads and wirelessly transmit this information to the receiver in the ICUMC. The ICUAC will use this data to build a continuous three-dimensional electrophysiological model of the patient's beating heart, constantly evaluating the myocardium for adequate perfusion and signal conduction. These same sensors will transmit the sounds made as ventilation gas flows through the bronchial tree into the small airways of the patient's lungs. The passive vibration of each inspiration and exhalation will be converted by complex software into a dynamic image of the patient's lungs and thoracic viscera. Each breath will allow a sophisticated three-dimensional image of the patient's lungs, pleura, and mediastinum to be generated for continuous evaluation by the ICUAI and the patient's intensivists.

Interposed between the patient's endotracheal tube and the ventilator, a senor continually acquires Et_{CO2}, V_{CO2}, V_{O2}, Vti, Vte, airway resistance, alveolar ventilation, minute volume, circuit and airway dead space, shunting, dynamic compliance, mean airway pressure, peak inspiratory and expiratory flow rates, work of breathing (WOB), and positive end expiratory pressure (PEEP). The ICUMC will integrate V_{O2} and V_{CO2} to determine resting energy expenditure (REE) and respiratory quotient (RQ). These parameters are continuously acquired by the ICUAI, evaluated, and used to update and shape the treatment algorithms. The transport team verifies the functioning of the ventilation profile sensor array, disconnects it from the ventilator in the ICU, and connects the sensor and the patient to the ICUMC ventilator tubing. The ventilation profile assembly is snapped onto yet another sensor in the ventilator circuit, the e-nose sensor array.

The e-nose microsensor array will relentlessly search for over a 200 chemicals looking for "smellprints" that will identify emerging infections — not only pneumonia or other pulmonary infections — but also systemic infections and free radical adducts. The senpA similar sensor array is present in the fecal management tube that the ICU transport team places in the patient's rectum. This sensor will provide surveillance of feces for both essential and undesirable gut flora and evaluate fecal matter for metabolites and nutrient absorption. After the balloon on the fecal management tubes is inflated, the team cleans and disinfects the patient's perineum thoroughly. The fecal management tube will serve the important function of preventing contamination of the patient's wounds with gut flora, prevent local irritation and skin breakdown, and decrease the burden of care on staff.

The team evaluates the integrity of the many in vivo sensors before transferring the patient to the ICUMC. Aortic root and central venous sensors placed during resuscitation and stabilization efforts in the ambulance were still in place and functioning. This new generation of monitors returns a staggering array of physiological data. All electrolytes, blood gases, pH, and saturations are continuously acquired from a series of sensors each about 50 microns in diameter strung out along a catheter 400 microns in diameter (roughly three times the diameter of a human hair). The fiber sensor array terminates in three unfurled kites; each a microsensor array with the capability of identifying and dynamically reporting the levels of over 100 different molecules. These two sensor arrays report the levels of myriads of biochemicals including cytokines modulating immunity, signaling molecules used by pathogenic bacterial, markers of injury released by damaged cells, and more than 100 other signaling molecules which initiate or modulate both cell repair and destruction.

The surgical team parenchymally in multiple areas of the lungs, myocardium, liver, and gut placed similar sensor arrays. Both the intravascular and parenchymal in vivo sensors terminate in two small buttons on the patient's skin: transmitters that relay the huge mass of data collected to the ICUAI via the ICUMC.

The patient had been transferred from the operating table to the critical care module (CCM) in the OR. Once instrumented, data began streaming from the sensor arrays on and in Herr van der Groot, to the hospital's central AI center and to the ICU's slave AI (ICUAI). As the patient arrived, Dr. Shen Shuang was joined by the neurointensivist Dr. Kong Tu and the patient's critical care nurse (CCRN) Jun Ge. Nurse Ge began connecting the patient's intravenous ports to the fluid pack assembled by the ICUAI and Drs. Shuang and Tu began working with the ICUAI to perform the admitting exam and initialize the patient's formal care plan.

ICUAI, speaking, as always, in its calm but authoritative voice, began working with the physicians by reporting on the patient's systems status and reviewing the standard algorithm-driven care that had already been initiated. Mechanical ventilation was proceeding at an Fi_{O2} of 0.8, PEEP of 10 cm H_2O, with the lung protective ventilation algorithm being used to determine tidal and minute volume. Over the next 15 minutes, a massive stream of data from the patient was integrated by the ICUAI and a prognosis and treatment plan was proposed to the physicians. The prognosis was extremely guarded. The ICUAI informed the treatment team that preliminary analysis of multiple species of injury marker molecules indicated very severe global injury to the liver parenchyma as well as rapidly evolving injury in the pulmonary parenchyma as well. The ICUAI suggested an interventional algorithm to moderate the patient's proinflammatory cascade that was already in the early stages of upregulating towards full-blown systemic inflammatory response syndrome (SIRS). While enormous progress had been made in salvaging patients such as Herr van der Groot, with more than 80% of such patients surviving with minimal or no lasting morbidity where none would have survived in the past, van der Groot's injuries were more serious than first thought. Furthermore, his genomic profile indicated that he was virtually certain to respond to this insult by turning off genes vital to moderating his inflammatory response and activating critical cellular repair systems. In particular, ICUAI reported that the patient had a genomic profile that resulted in severe, acute mitochondrial damage, particularly in hepatocytes. Significant progress had been made in modulating such adverse gene activity, but the state of the art was still far removed from routine control. A major complicating factor was the time required to perform genomic analysis and the rapidity of the free radical–mediated destruction of hepatic mitochondria in such susceptible patients.

Dr. Shuang and Dr. Tu decided on a treatment plan that would consist of aggressive homeostatic support, moderation of the immune inflammatory cascade (IIC), and organ function support/replacement limited to mechanical ventilation and renal replacement therapy (RRT). The physicians consulted the ICUAI for survival projections in the event of liver failure and determined that, given the magnitude of the polytrauma, the patient's genomics, and the rapidly evolving injury to the lungs that the patient was not a viable candidate for liver transplant (<less than> 2% chance of survival).

Two hours after his admission to the ICU, Dr. Shuang met with Herr van der Groot's next-of-kin, his father and brother, both of whom had been traveling with him. Dr. Shuang explained the patient's situation and prognosis and escorted the family to visit Herr van der Groot in the ICU. During this visit the patient's brother, Wilhem, asked where Herr van der Groot's emergency cryopreservation necktag was. Had the hospital staff removed it? Dr. Shuang indicated that he was unaware that Herr van der Groot had cryopreservation arrangements. While the practice was growing rapidly among the affluent in China, it was still very unusual and quite controversial in the West, with the practice being forbidden in almost half a dozen Western nations.

Wilhem explained that his brother Aschwin had made arrangements for cryopreservation in the event of his medicolegal death when he was in his early 20s, and had actually worked as a research assistant in the United States in the laboratory where the first parenchymatous mammalian organs (the kidney and the heart) had been successfully cryopreserved, leading the establishment of the worldwide organ cryobanking industry. While whole-body cryopreservation was still not possible, Aschwin van der Groot and his brother Wilhem both believed that viable cryogenic storage of the brain in a glassy, ice-free state known as vitrification offered the promise of rescue in the future by ever more rapidly advancing medical technology.

Cryopreservation organizations perfused their patients with a mixture of cryoprotectants optimized to allow essentially reversible cryopreservation of the brain. Constraints on cooling rate due the mass of the trunk and the peculiar requirements of some vital organs meant that the procedure could not be undertaken without causing some ice formation, particularly in tissues that are poorly circulated (such as the gut). Patients treated in this way would thus have potentially viable brains (in the absence of prior brain injury) but would need to await vast advances in medicine to repair damage to organs injured by both cryopreservation and currently irreversible disease. The idea had originated in the United States in the 1960s, but had been dogged by scientific skepticism, scandal, and serious legal challenges. By contrast, with the introduction of organ cryobanking into China in 2012, the practice had faced little resistance and rapidly became the most popular option for terminally ill Chinese patients who had the means to afford it.

Dr. Shuang quickly informed Dr. Tu and Nurse Ge of this new development. In consultation with ICUAI and the patient's family, the medical team decided on a treatment plan that would include discontinuation of conventional life support in the event the patient experienced multisystem organ failure with no acceptable chance of recovery, or in the event the patient developed any potentially irreversible neurological morbidity. In consultation with the Herr van der Groot's family and his prior directive concerning his medical care and cryopreservation arrangements downloaded from his e-records at the cryopresergvation company (a copy of which had been the jump drive/ID tag he wore around his neck), it was decided that if the probability of survival dropped below 10% as determined by the ICUAI algorithms and Dr. Shuang's and Tu's judgements, femoral bypass cannulae would be placed and mechanical ventilation and homeostatic support would be withdrawn at which time the patient would undergo blood washout with TransPlanned, a hypothermic organ preservation solution, and would be cooled to ~2°C for transfer to the cryopreservation organization.

During the next 48 hours Herr van der Groot's condition followed the trajectory anticipated by the ICUAI. After seeming to rally initially, and even regain consciousness, both liver and lung function began to deteriorate relentlessly. While the patient's kidneys continued to function, the patient's hepatocytes became progressively dysfunctuional and necrotic. Pulmonary edema, present from the time patient was admitted to hospital, grew progressively worse with the SV_{O2} declining to 55% at an Fi_{O2} of 1.0. During his brief period of consciousness, the patient was told of his prognosis and indicated his strong desire to be cryopreserved for future rescue.

At 1045 on the third day of his stay in ICU the ICUAI alerted the treating medical staff that the patient's condition and prognosis now met the criteria for cryopreservation. Dr. Kong Tu was on duty when this alert was issued and summoned the patient's family to allow them to say their goodbyes. Following this "final" family visit, the patient was percutaneously cannulated for femoral–femoral bypass. The patient was perfused with cold, oxygenated TransPlanned preservation solution with progressive hemodilution as his core temperature rapidly descended toward 0°C. Cardiac arrest occurred as the temperature passed through +18°C. As was customary for cryopreservation patients, this was recorded as the time of death, even though TransPlanned was known to sustain life for up 7 hours of asanguineous perfusion at near freezing temperatures without neurological deficit. This would be more than enough time to transport Herr van der Groot to the Shanghai cryopreservation facility that had a cooperative agreement with his cryopreservation company.

Upon arrival at the cryoprepreservation facility, cold perfusion was stopped for 30 minutes while the percutaneous cannulae were replaced with large bore femoral cannula suitable for perfusion of viscous solutions. At a temperature of +3°C, the neurological consequences of this period of circulatory arrest would be minimal. Perfusion was resumed with a gradually increasing concentration of cryoprotectant chemicals that prevent freezing by binding and replacing water molecules inside cells. As the cryoprotectant concentration increased, and the perfusate melting point decreased, the perfusion temperature was lowered to reduce toxic effects of the water replacement process. This process mirrored methods developed to prepare transplantable organs for long-term banking at cryogenic temperatures. Cryoprotectant perfusion ended 4 hours after it began. The patient was now at a temperature of −30°C, but with 70% of the water inside his body replaced by cryoprotectant molecules that made freezing impossible in many tissues. Rather than freezing, molecules would just move slower and slower as temperature decreased, maintaining normal structural integrity of cells and tissues.

The final phase of the process consisted of placing the patient in a stream of cold nitrogen gas that would cool his core to a temperature of $-115°C$ within 5 hours, and then further to $-140°C$ over 4 weeks. At that temperature, well below the glass transition temperature of $-125°C$, Aschwin van der Groot would exist in a glassy solid state (vitrification) in which biological time was stopped. Although in this state he will still be neurologically viable and recoverable by contemporary technology, numerous injuries to other vital systems and tissues, including sensory organs, would preclude any meaningful recovery until technologies for comprehensive tissue and organ regeneration were available. On that basis cryopreservation patients were considered dead, although this was becoming increasingly controversial.

Back at Zhongshan Hospital, Dr. Shuang wondered if he had ever see Herr van der Groot again. While he himself is 40 years old, with a remaining life expectancy of 60 more years, it is hard for him to imagine the required developments coming to fruition in his lifetime. While thousands of people were beginning to bet on what the ultimate limits of medicine might be, he is still painfully aware of what those limits are today.

References

1. Drexler KE. Engines of creation. New York: Doubleday; 1986. Available at: http://www.foresight.org/EOC/EOC_Chapter_3.html#section04of05.
2. Binnig G, Rohrer H, et al. Tunneling through a controllable vacuum gap. Appl Phys Lett 1982;40:178–180.
3. Drexler KE. Nanosystems: molecular machinery, manufacturing, and computation. New York: Wiley Interscience; 1992.
4. Sapsford KE, Soto CM, et al. A cowpea mosaic virus nanoscaffold for multiplexed antibody conjugation: application as an immunoassay tracer. Biosens Bioelectron 2005;21:1668–1673.
5. Lin T, Johnson, JE, et al. Structure-based engineering of an icosahedral virus for nanomedicine and nanotechnology. The Scripps Institute Scientific Report. La Jolla, CA: Scripps Institute; 2004.
6. Clarke AC. Peacetime uses for V-2; V-2 for ionosphere research? Wireless World. February1945:58.
7. Thomas L. Lives of a cell. New York: Viking Press; 1974:299.
8. Halpern NA, Pastores SM, Greenstein RJ. Critical care medicine in the United States 1985-2000: an analysis of bed numbers, use, and costs. Crit Care Med 2004;32:1408–1409.
9. Chalfin DB, Cohen IL, Lanken PN. The economics and cost-effectiveness of critical care medicine. Intensive Care Med 1995;21:952–961.
10. Lee R, Tuljapurkar S. Death and taxes: longer life, consumption, and social security. Demography 1997;34:67–81.
11. de Grey ADNJ, Ames BN, et al. Time to talk SENS: critiquing the immutability of human aging. Ann N Y Acad Sci 2002;959:452–462.

12. Hayflick L. How and why we age. Westminister, MD: Ballantine Books; 1996.
13. Holmes OW. The one horse shay and its companion poems. Cambridge, MA: Houghton, Mifflin and Company, The Riverside Press; 1892.
14. Kurzweil R. The law of accelerating returns. Available at: http://www.kurzweilai.net/articles/art0134.html?printable=1.
15. Becker GS. Get the FDA out of the way, and drug prices will drop. Business Week. September 16, 2002:16.
16. The Cato Institute Handbook for the 105th Congress. Section 32. Washington, DC: Cato Institute; 1997. Available at: http://www.cato.org/pubs/handbook/hb105-32.html.
17. Smith P. Arrows of mercy. Toronto: Doubleday; 1969:178.
18. Lindsay J. Harold Griffiths and the introduction of curare. J Can Med Assoc 1991;144:588–589.
19. Meyer JA. Werner Forssman and cardiac catherterization of the heart. Ann Thorac Surg 1990;49:497–499.
20. Gott VL. King of hearts: the true story of the maverick who pioneered open heart surgery. New York: Crown Publishers; 2000.
21. Pietzman SJ. Chronic dialysis and dialysis doctors in the United States: a nephrologist-historian's perspective. Semin Dialysis 2001;14:200–208.
22. Dialysis Corporation of America Annual Report (10-K) for Dec 31, 2004.
23. Committee on Metabolic Monitoring for Military Field Applications, Standing Committee on Military Nutrition Research. Monitoring metabolic status: predicting decrements in physiological and cognitive performance. Washington, DC: National Academy Press; 2004.

Afterword

David W. Crippen

> Imagination is the beginning of creation. You imagine
> what you desire, you will what you imagine and at last
> you create what you will.
>
> —George Bernard Shaw

This is a treatise on how the emerging global community deals with some facets of healthcare delivery — specifically, intensive care. The reader will discern many similarities in the way in which health care is delivered in the global village and how financing figures into that care. One of the most striking similarities, occurring in most developed countries, is that some form of healthcare coverage is provided for the entire population. The United States is the only developed country that excludes a portion of its citizens from health care, for reasons that remain unclear.

Other factions of the global medical community recognize and accept that some prioritization is needed to spread resources through an entire population. With such an approach, some restrictions and waiting are necessary for the system to meet demand. Americans have become accustomed to an entitlement system. The best insured get highest priority. To facilitate that culture, only part of the population receives facilitated service. The fortunate receive health insurance through employment or through government plans (for those older than 65). Others rely on inadequate benefits from welfare schemes or have no medical benefits at all.

In 2006, between 51.2 million and 53.7 million Americans will be excluded from health insurance by one means or another,[1] an increase of 10 million from the last 5 years. More than 70% of the uninsured live in families with at least one full-time worker.[2] Workers who can afford insurance have as much as an 8.5% payroll deduction,[3] a number that is increasing by about 14% per year. The last annual hike in health insurance premiums mostly paid by employers (12.7%) is more than five times the increase in 1998. The average premium for employer-sponsored family health coverage will surge to US $14,545 in 2006, double the average premium in 2001.[4]

The latest figures show that the United States is currently spending well over 15.6% of its gross national product on health care[5] — up 9.3% in 10 years, to a total of US $1.55 trillion, or an average of $5,440 for each person in the United States. Hospital care and prescription drugs outstripped the rest of the country's growth for the fourth year in a row, with no end in sight. Employers are finding it difficult or impossible to continue financing employee health benefits and are cutting back those benefits.[6]

Many reasons have been offered for this quandary of high-cost, low-efficiency medical care. One is the curious practice of "path of least resistance" reimbursement. Almost 20% of our population is denied access to many early preventive measures. These individuals finally do enter the healthcare pipeline, usually through emergency facilities, and the system must still pay for their care. It is a myth that we are saving money by not providing care to a portion of our population, thus enabling us to expend those saved resources on others. In the end, they all end up in the same place, but by circuitous routes that increase expense by increasing inefficiency, and the healthcare system is collapsing under the weight. Between 1995 and 1997, 3% of hospitals closed and 5.8% merged; between 1998 and 2000, 3.2% closed and 2.2% merged.[7] Although American health care is the most expensive, the United States is not among the top 40 countries in terms of quality of care (as measured by life expectancy), according to the World Health Organization.[8]

This sociopolitical conundrum of rising costs, dubious quality, and decreasing availability directly affects the most expensive use of scarce resources, intensive care. This treatise, authored by an eclectic selection of global providers of critical care, seeks to compare and contrast similarities and differences in the emerging global standard of care. The following question was asked: If there are differences, why do they exist, and are they departures from a global mean that has evolved for greatest efficiency or are they simply extraneous regional variations?

One feature that separates the American healthcare system from the healthcare systems of the rest of the global medical community is autonomy. The global maxim is to restrict immediate gratification of some to support long-term goals for all. The American attitude is that health care is a basic right and should be available to all on demand. And the fundamental principle of autonomy demands that patients and their families have a hand in medical decisions made by physicians.

The interpretation of patient autonomy in American health care, however, is curiously inconsistent. For example, patients and their families can and do demand intensive care even when it is judged to carry no benefit. But a surgeon does not have to perform an operation he or she believes is of no benefit just because the patient demands it, and a patient has no right to demand chemotherapy that an oncologist deems useless. What is the basis for these seemingly divergent interpretations of autonomy? The key concept is the avoidance of paternalism in the expenditure of scarce resources. The supposition is that providers have no right to interfere with the desires of patients and their families and ought not even to ask for justification, lest they raise the specter of discrimination. Once justification is asked for, it is easy to manipulate possible justifications to suit the biases of providers.

The global village is remarkably consistent in its standard for providing effective intensive care to critically ill patients. It is when there is disparity in opinions regarding prioritization that there is divergence. In the global village, some individual autonomy is subjugated to support a greater good. In the United States, however, patients and their families sometimes demand unrealistic care on the basis of unrealistic expectations, and when a long-shot miracle is awaited, open-ended pain and suffering can result. Why does this paradox between palliation and tribulation exist? Several answers have been suggested for the American geography of the global village:

- Physicians do not have an exceptional track record in explaining end-of-life issues to patients and their families, and many do not understand the concept themselves.[9] The current notion of medical futility as an end-stage process in which vital signs cannot be supported further is poorly understood by both physicians and surrogates.[10] They approach end of life as either all black or all white. They consider that the options for care at the end of life are only two: everything or nothing. Given that choice, most surrogates opt for doing something rather than nothing, even if the former perpetuates open-ended pain and discomfort (masked by sedation). Providers fail to communicate that there is a third option, that of maintaining aggressive treatment but switching to comfort measures if some knockout blow occurs, rather than prolonging the dying process.

- Because of the competitive nature of medical practice in America, especially private practice, which thrives in community hospital centers, physicians have a strong incentive to promote customer satisfaction. The airlines say: "We know you have a choice in your air travel, and we're pleased you chose us." Likewise, patients with a choice tend to choose physicians who satisfy their desires. This puts patients in the position of being buyers in a competitive consumer market. Physicians outline choices for them but are reluctant to be bearers of bad news. In essence, physicians tell patients that they, the patients, have the authority to choose. In this manner, physicians imply that patients' authority to make choices extends to making bad choices.

- Before the advent of critical care, patients sent signals concerning their degree of health, discomfort, and survivability. Patients who looked bad were bad. These signals resonated with their surrogates. However, most moribund patients on life support in an intensive care unit (ICU) look comfortable. An observer's primal reaction to the vibrant external appearance of a body supported in an ICU is radically different from a reaction to the appearance of a corpse on a morgue slab.[11] As long as the patient looks "viable," it is easier to accept the premise that there is enhanced survivability; it is easier to believe that if the patient can just be maintained comfortably long enough, he or she may be cured.

- Surrogates are uncomfortable when asked to make decisions that directly result in the death of a loved one. The phrase *withdrawing life support* directly implies promoting death by decanting life. Life-in-death can be a much more palatable alternative to death if the patient appears comfortable and death can be postponed indefinitely.

- The popular media, especially the tabloids, frequently present stories of individuals who have awakened after years of indolent "coma.[12]" Most, if not all, of these patients' conditions have been embellished to generate public interest, and subsequent investigators frequently cannot find these patients. After hearing such stories, some families think that if life-support systems can maintain vital signs for a day or a week, suspended animation should be possible indefinitely, until a cure is found.

A fundamental global question remains: Under what circumstances should patients and their families have the authority to trump providers' differing opinions on benefit? The experience of the global community suggests that any differences between providers and surrogates regarding ICU end-of-life issues can be mediated by continuing dialogue.[3] The ethos of these discussions, however, varies in different parts of the global village (Stephen Streat, personal communication). The differentiation between consensus and consent is a major point of divergence. For example, critical care physicians in New Zealand strive for "consensus without consent"(Tim Buchman, personal communication). Discussions with surrogates strive for concordance and understanding but do not extend to solicitation of consent for medically inappropriate care. New Zealand physicians simply do not offer inappropriate end-of-life care. But in America, consensus must necessarily include consent, and so if an impasse is reached, patient and surrogate wishes are frequently followed as a matter of policy.

As of this writing, no meaningful resolution to this dilemma has been reached, and the global village continues to struggle with the consequences. Fundamental questions about how to finance the maintenance of warm cadavers in the ICU are politically taboo and simply not addressed. The issue of supporting a 99% probability of continued pain and suffering because of a 1% probability of benefit at some time in the future is socially taboo and not addressed. Embracing paternalism portends a far worse ethical calamity than any of the above, and we are content to pay for it in occult currency. Americans will eventually deal with these issues, but we will put off doing so as long as possible. Perhaps the vision of the global village will show us the way.

This volume could not have been completed without the miracle of the Internet, which has brought critical care physicians together like never before. The Internet made possible this book's exploration of critical care in the global village. It is our sincere hope that the global expertise represented here will result in continued growth in learning and knowledge.

Special thanks to Mike Darwin, whose visions and perceptions are superhuman and who I hope will someday drink a glass of wine while sitting on one of Saturn's rings; and to Leslie Whetstine, one of the new breed of medical ethicists who will change the world. Thanks also to the doctors and paramedical professionals of the global village. Our time has come.

References

1. Available at: http://www.cdc.gov/nchs/.
2. Available at: http://democrats.house.gov/bigpicture/health/.

3. Thorpe KE. The National Coalition on Health Care specifications for reform: impacts on health care spending and federal costs. Available at: http://www.nchc.org/materials/nchcpressclub-final%20copy.pdf. Accessed May 8, 2006.

4. Simmons HE, Goldberg MA. Charting the cost of inaction. Washington, DC: National Coalition on Health Care; 2003.

5. Rising health care costs force employers to cut some non-essential benefits: SHRM releases its 2003 survey of employer benefits. Available at: http://www.business-knowhow.com/manage/hccosts.htm. Accessed May 8, 2006.

6. Available at: http://www.os.dhhs.gov/.

7. Bazzoli G. America's hospitals: in danger or bouncing back [text version of slide presentation]? Available at: http://www.ahcpr.gov/news/ulp/hospital/bazzolitxt.htm. Accessed May 8, 2006.

8. Available at: http://www.nationmaster.com/.

9. Lynn J, Teno JM, Phillips RS, et al. Perceptions by family members of the dying experience of older and seriously ill patients. SUPPORT Investigators. Study to Understand Prognoses and Preferences for Outcomes and Risks of Treatments. Ann Intern Med 1997;126:97–106.

10. Frick S, Uehlinger DE, Zuercher Zenklusen RM. Medical futility: predicting outcome of intensive care unit patients by nurses and doctors—a prospective comparative study. Crit Care Med 2003;31:456–461.

11. Whetstine L. When is "dead" dead: an examination of the medical and philosophical literature on the determination of death [dissertation]. Pittsburgh, PA: Duquesne University; 2004.

12. Man awakes after 19 years in coma. Available at: http://www.cbsnews.com/stories/2003/07/09/health/main562293.shtml. Accessed May 8, 2006.

13. Crippen D, Kilcullen JK, Kelly DF, eds. Three patients: international perspective on intensive care at the end of life. Boston: Kluwer Academic Publishers; 2002.

Index